Issues in Aging
(Vol. 7)
Garland Reference Library of Social Science
(Vol. 983)

Issues in Aging

Diana K. Harris, Series Editor

The Remainder of Their Days
Domestic Policy and Older Families in the United States and Canada
edited by Jon Hendricks and Carolyn J. Rosenthal

Housing and the Aging Population
Options for the New Century
edited by W. Edward Folts and Dale E. Yeatts

Services to the Aging and Aged
Public Policies and Programs
edited by Paul K.H. Kim

The Political Behavior of Older Americans
edited by Steven A. Peterson and Albert Somit

Aging in the Twenty-first Century
A Developmental Perspective
edited by Len Sperry and Harry Prosen

Part-Time Employment for the Low-Income Elderly
Experiences from the Field
by Leslie B. Alexander and Lenard W. Kaye

Men Giving Care
Reflections of Husbands and Sons
by Phyllis Braudy Harris and Joyce Bichler

Men Giving Care
Reflections of Husbands and Sons

Phyllis Braudy Harris
Joyce Bichler

GARLAND PUBLISHING, INC.
New York & London
1997

Library of Congress Cataloging-in-Publication Data

Harris, Phyllis Braudy.
        Men giving care : reflections of husbands and sons / Phyllis
Braudy Harris, Joyce Bichler.
                p.   cm. — (Garland reference library of social science ;
vol. 983. Issues in aging ; vol. 7)
        Includes bibliographical references and index.
        ISBN 0-8153-1792-1 (alk. paper)
                1. Aged—Care—United States—Case studies.   2. Alzheimer's
disease—Patients—Care—United States—Case studies.   3. Caregivers—United States—Case studies.   4. Husbands—United States—
Case studies.   5. Sons—United States—Case studies.   I. Bichler,
Joyce. II. Title.   III. Series: Garland reference library of social
science ; vol. 983.   IV. Series: Garland reference library of social
science. Issues in aging; v. 7.
        HV1461.H39   1997
        362.1'96831—DC21   96–48449
                                                                                    CIP

Printed on acid-free, 250-year-life paper
Manufactured in the United States of America

Contents

Series Editor's Preface   vii

Acknowledgments   ix

Introduction   xi

Chapter One
Caring for an Elderly Family Member   1
Changing Patterns?

Part One: Husbands as Caregivers
Their Inner World

Chapter Two
**Husbands' Characteristics, Common Themes,
and Shared Experiences**   17

Chapter Three
Toward a Typology of Husband Caregivers   35

Chapter Four
Husbands   73
Service Implications—What Can We Learn?

Part Two: Sons as Caregivers
Their Inner World

Chapter Five
**Sons' Characteristics, Common Themes,
and Shared Experiences**   91

Chapter Six
Toward a Typology of Son Caregivers   111

Chapter Seven
Sons   159
Service Implications—What Can We Learn?

Chapter Eight
Contrasts, Questions, and Final Reflections   169

Appendices

Appendix A
Interview Guides for Husband and Son Caregivers   179

Appendix B
Characteristics of Husband and Son Caregivers   183

Appendix C
Early Stage Programs   187

Appendix D
Computer Support Networks   191

Appendix E
Hiring In-Home Help   193

Appendix F
Evaluating Adult Day Care Services   205

Appendix G
Alzheimer's Care in Residential Settings   209

Appendix H
A Sample Care Management Program   213

References   217
Index   221

Series Editor's Preface

This series attempts to address the topic of aging from a wide variety of perspectives and to make available some of the best gerontological thought and writing to researchers, professional practitioners, and students in the field of aging as well as in other related areas. All the volumes in the series are written and/or edited by outstanding scholars and leading specialists on current issues of considerable interest.

Men Giving Care: Reflections of Husbands and Sons uses data drawn from interviews with husbands and sons who care for their wives and parents with dementia. In their own words, these men describe their lives and experiences as informal caregivers. Their narratives are insightful, informative, and provocative. Clearly and concisely written, this book makes a valuable contribution and is a welcome addition to the sparse literature on male caregivers.

Diana K. Harris
The University of Tennessee

Acknowledgments

First and foremost we want to express our appreciation and gratitude to the 30 husbands and 30 sons who let us into their homes and lives. They unhesitatingly answered our questions and shared with us their narratives about caring for a wife or parent with dementia. Their words make this book come to life. From their experiences our understanding of the role of the male caregiver has been enhanced. We are grateful for the unwavering support from the Cleveland Area Alzheimer's Association. Casey Durkin, Sharen Eckert, and Sally Ollerton were invaluable advisors, and they also assisted us in recruiting male caregivers for the study.

This book would not be possible without the painstaking work of our tape transcriber, Karen Rocco. The hours she spent and the outstanding caliber of her work in transcribing the interviews is evident throughout the book. A special word of thanks goes to our colleagues and friends Susan Long, Marcia Neundorfer, and Patti Gibson for reading various versions of the manuscript and providing detailed comments that improved the quality of the book. Also Diana Harris, editor of Garland's Issues in Aging series, continually provided words of encouragement.

Finally to our husbands, Jim Harris and Michael Kimbarow, we give our heartfelt thanks. Their humor, perspectives, constructive criticism, and belief in us helped carry us throughout the writing process. Phyllis especially wants to thank her two sons, Dan and Jeff, whose patience, understanding, and support went far beyond their young years.

This research was supported in part by grants from the Cleveland Foundation and John Carroll University.

Introduction

Upon leaving a board meeting of the local chapter of the Alzheimer's Association, I found myself on the elevator with two elderly board members. Between them they had over 16 years of experience caring for their wives who had Alzheimer's disease. As there were only the three of us in the elevator, I could not help overhearing their conversation. It went something like this:

How's your wife doing?

Things are about the same. Her condition hasn't changed much in the last year. That's about all I can hope for now. I have set up a hospital bed in my living room so I can be nearer to her during the day. I still work part-time, and I have someone coming in to help me, but it's those evening hours that are the hardest. When I come home from work, not having anyone to share my thoughts with, or to tell about my day, or to help me with those day-to-day decisions we always made together, and then . . . having to eat another night of my own cooking. . . .

I know how you feel. I'm home by myself now. I had to place my wife in a nursing home; it's the hardest thing I ever had to do. I visit my wife twice a day to help feed her and then I come home to an empty house. . . . But I do have this wonderful and easy steak recipe.

As the elevator doors opened and I walked out, I left these two men sharing recipes.

The next day in my office at the university, I continued working on a paper I was presenting, but I couldn't get the image and conversation of these two elderly gentlemen out of my mind.

I began to notice how few studies had been done on male caregivers. The studies that have been done suggest that, compared to women, men experience less emotional distress, feel less burden due to the demands of caregiving, have higher morale, and provide less hands-on care (e.g., Fitting et al., 1986; Horowitz, 1985; Gilhooly, 1984; Pruchno & Resch, 1989; Young & Kahana, 1989; George, 1984). This seemed at odds with the conversation I had heard the night before.

I reflected on conversations I had with other male caregivers, husbands and sons, in clinical settings, educational workshops, and informal gatherings. Again, there seemed to be a discrepancy between what these men told me and what the research reported. I decided an in depth study was needed on male caregivers to allow these men to relate their experiences in their own words. The insights gained from these conversations would contribute a deeper understanding of what it is like for a man to be caring for a wife or parent with severe memory loss. It also could provide assistance for family members, clinicians, educators, program planners, researchers, and policymakers.

My first step was to solicit the help of the Cleveland Area Chapter of the Alzheimer's Association. Their research review board and patient-family advisory committees approved and strongly endorsed my proposed research. The program staff worked diligently to provide me easy access to their population of male caregivers. In the process of working with the Alzheimer's Association, I also gained a new advocate for the men, the then program director and now co-author of this book, Joyce Bichler, M.S.W. Joyce's enthusiasm and helpful suggestions made me realize the benefit of having someone with her clinical expertise involved in writing this book.

Our strengths complement each other. My strength is in the area of research and education, and Joyce's is in program planning and advocacy. By bringing our common interests and our different strengths together, our goal is to bridge that often shaky connection between research and practice. We hope that together we can ensure that the voices of these male caregivers will be heard.

As I am the originator of the study and the researcher of the book, we decided that I would take the major responsibility for writing, except for the practice sections, where Joyce would be the lead author. The book as a whole, however, is a cooperative effort, with each of us discussing, critiquing, and editing each other's work. It has developed into a true joint venture.

The book is divided into two major parts, the first on husbands and the second on sons, with Chapter 1 providing background for both parts. Chapter 1 gives a brief description of previous research on husbands and sons as caregivers. It also describes the method used to gather information for this study from the 60 men interviewed and outlines the four research questions that guided the study: (1) What is it like for a man to take on a major caregiving role? (2) How does he adapt to and cope with his new functions? (3) What are his motivations for taking on this role? and (4) What, if any, meaning does he derive from this caregiving experience?

Part I starts with Chapter 2 and focuses on the lives of husbands caring for wives with severe memory loss. The main cause of this memory loss was Alzheimer's disease, though there were other related disorders that caused the same symptoms. This chapter describes the husbands who participated in the study and identifies and examines the common experiences discussed by husband caregivers. The men express in their own words their motivations, concerns, issues, struggles, and achievements as they care for their wives. Chapter 3 focuses on the different ways in which these men have adapted to their new role of caring for a wife with memory loss. A typology of five types of husband caregivers is identified. Each of these five types has its own predominant characteristics and behaviors that aid in the caregiving process. We provide narratives of 14 husbands' caregiving experiences to demonstrate these different orientations. Chapter 4 concludes the section on husband caregivers by presenting practice implications based on the husbands' perspectives. Helpful programs and services the husbands have used are reviewed, and suggestions for new needed services for male caregivers are proposed.

Part II centers on the lives of sons as they care for mothers or fathers, and sometimes both, who have severe memory loss. This section follows the same format as the previous section: Chapter 5 describes the sons who participated in the study and also focuses on their commonalities and shared experiences, using their own words; Chapter 6 discusses ways in which the sons have oriented themselves to their caregiver roles and identifies with examples four types of son caregivers; and Chapter 7 presents service and program suggestions from the sons' perspectives. It also highlights similarities to and differences from the husbands' recommendations.

The book concludes with Chapter 8, which discusses some of the contrasts and similarities in the caregiving experiences of sons and husbands, and considers racial and social class differences across all the caregivers. We review the original four research questions that guided the study and discuss how the information from the interviews with these 60 men moves us a step closer to answering these questions. We also propose other questions about male caregivers that still need to be considered.

Our hope is that by the conclusion of this book, readers will have entered the world of the male caregiver. They will have heard their voices, shared their reflections, and, consequently, gained some understanding of their experiences. The two men in the elevator who inspired this research represent much more than two men with ill wives sharing recipes. They reflect a piece of the caregiving experience of each man in this study and in doing so mirror their commitment, despair, pain, love, dilemmas, hardships, rewards, satisfactions, and hopes.

Phyllis Braudy Harris, Ph.D.
John Carroll University
Cleveland, Ohio
July 1995

Men Giving Care

Chapter One
Caring for an Elderly Family Member
Changing Patterns?

The family has always been the primary source of care for an elderly relative in the United States, and it continues to be so today. This has been well documented in the gerontological literature of the past 30 years (Shanas and Strieb, 1965; Shanas, 1979; Cantor, 1983; U.S. Senate Special Committee on Aging, 1987). Despite this longstanding trend, we still are periodically bombarded with sensational newspaper articles and television news reports about families that abandon their ill elderly. The day-to-day care of sick elderly family members does not make exciting news.

Traditionally, the bulk of caring for the elderly has fallen on women, mainly wives and daughters, and of that there can be no dispute (Horowitz, 1985; Brody, 1990; Abel, 1991). Women have always been involved in the hands-on day-to-day care of impaired husbands and parents. Even in the last two decades, with women entering the work force in unparalleled numbers, their level of involvement and commitment to caring for the elderly has not faltered or changed (Brody et al., 1987; Scharlach, Lowe, and Schneider, 1991). Yet there are also men involved in providing care to their elderly family members, going against the traditionally accepted roles. There are fewer male caregivers than female, but they appear to be just as committed (Motenko, 1988; Harris, 1993). What do we know about these caregivers? The next section focuses on these men.

What about the Male Caregiver?
Although gender roles have been studied as an issue in caregiving since the early 1980s, it wasn't until recently that researchers adjusted the focus of their studies to include men in the caregiving role (Kaye and Applegate, 1990a, 1990b). And, as often happens when

one is trying to adjust the focus and examine a new phenomenon, the findings are often blurred and at times contradictory.

The exact percentage of male caregivers varies, depending upon the study. In a study by Stone, Cafferata, and Sangl (1987), based on the 1982 National Long-Term Care Survey and Informal Caregivers Survey, male caregivers were estimated to compose 28 percent of all caregivers, with husbands constituting the largest group, 13 percent. In a study by the American Association of Retired Persons and Travelers Foundation, it was estimated that 25 percent of the seven million elderly caregivers are men (Weinstein, 1989). In another study done by Louis Harris and Associates for the Commonwealth Fund (1993), which included men aged 55 and older, 20 percent of the caregivers were men. According to all three studies, at least one-quarter of all caregivers are men. The number of male caregivers is expected to grow as the elderly population lives longer.

Most of the research on male caregivers has concentrated on husbands, who make up the majority of male caregivers. Studies on husband caregivers have shown some consistent findings as well as many contradictions. Some of the consistent conclusions regarding husband caregivers center around issues of commitment, control, and mental health. Spouses—husbands as well as wives—provide the most consistent and dependable care for longer periods of time than any other caregivers (Johnson, 1983; Doty, 1986; Stoller, 1992). A husband's commitment to caring for an impaired wife is a theme that is echoed in much of the research (Motenko, 1988; Harris, 1993). Some husbands feel comfortable in taking control of their wife's caregiving, an extension of their work role. As a matter of fact, this caregiving often becomes an new career (Miller, 1987, 1990; Harris, 1993). Other studies suggest that men fare better emotionally than women on a number of indicators of mental health. Men report lower caregiver burden (Horowitz, 1985; Fitting et al., 1986; Young and Kahana, 1989; Miller and Cafasso, 1992; Mui, 1995), although other researchers suggest this may be due to men's reluctance to complain and their need to "hang tough" (Horowitz, 1992; Barer, 1994). Husband caregivers also report higher morale (Gilhooly, 1984) and less psychotropic drug use (George, 1984).

There are, however, many contradictions in the sparse literature on male caregivers. Some studies examined coping strategies and found that husbands pursue their caring tasks with a problem-solving approach carried over from work roles (Zarit, 1982; Miller, 1987). Other studies did not find this stereotypic gender-role coping strategy (Borden and Berlin, 1990). Some studies found men were more likely than women to receive both informal and formal caregiving assistance in caring for their wives (Zarit, Todd, and Zarit, 1986; Johnson, 1983; Stone, Cafferata, and Sangl, 1987). Yet, other studies describe husbands' pride in their ability to manage on their own, to the point of not wanting assistance from their children (Vinick, 1984; Monteko, 1988; Harris, 1993). Some findings reveal that husbands in their new caregiving role felt closer to their wives and had improved relationships, for they felt needed by their wives and more involved than ever (Fitting et al., 1986; Motenko, 1988). However, other studies found that the quality of the relationship deteriorated, and tensions increased as the wives became less able to be companions and confidants (Wright, 1991; George and Gwyther, 1986).

Thus, the information we know so far about husbands is limited and sometimes confusing. More research on husbands caring for wives is needed, particularly research that emphasizes an in-depth understanding of the world of husband caregivers. Questions need to be asked that delve deeper into their experiences, such as: What is it like to be caring for a wife with progressive memory loss? How do husbands adapt? What are their motivations? What meaning do husbands give to this experience? Much more needs to be known.

The research on son caregivers is even sparser and more narrowly directed than the research on husbands. Although sons do not constitute the majority of the caregivers, one study of family caregivers estimates that they compose 10.8 percent of the total primary caregivers and 52.2 percent of the secondary caregivers to the elderly (Stone, Cafferata, and Sangl, 1987). In another study, based on a stratified random sample of elderly community dwellers, sons were estimated to comprise 12.4 percent of primary caregivers to frail elderly parents (Tennstedt, McKinlay, and Sullivan, 1989).

The few studies that have examined the role of son caregivers concentrated on the tasks performed by sons. Findings from these studies support gender stereotypes. Horowitz (1985) found in her sample of 32 sons that sons became caregivers only in the absence of available female caregivers; that they were more likely than daughters to rely on the support of their spouse; and that they provided less overall assistance, especially hands-on assistance, to their parents. Sons, though, are just as likely as daughters to provide financial and emotional support to their parents and to share their home with a parent. Montgomery and Kamo (1987) and Stoller (1992) found that sons provided intermittent assistance but were less involved in routine household chores. As the parents' level of functioning worsened over time, sons dropped out of the caregiving role. Dwyer and Coward's (1991) large multivariate comparison of 13,000 sons and daughters caring for impaired parents substantiates the above findings related to gender differences in caregiver tasks.

One study, though, did suggest a reason other than gender related behavior for daughters' predominance in the caregiving arena. The researchers proposed that children tend to feel more comfortable providing care to parents of the same sex as themselves. Because women generally have a longer life span than men, the number of male elderly to be cared for is less, and sons are not as comfortable as daughters in providing care to their mothers. This in turn leads to a smaller number of son caregivers (Lee, Dwyer, and Coward, 1993).

The above research illustrates differences between sons and daughters as caregivers, but does not provide us with an understanding of son caregivers. In order to obtain a clearer picture of sons in this role we need to ask such questions as: Why do they take on this untraditional gender role? What is it like for them? What does this role mean to them? How do they adapt? More in-depth research on sons is needed that goes beyond differences in tasks performed so we can gain a better understanding of the experiences of sons as caregivers to elderly parents. Like the information on husband caregivers, much is yet to be known.

The Changing Context of Male Caregiving

Caregiving by husbands and sons takes place against a background of changing patterns, gender and demographic. There is much debate about whether men in the 1990s are truly becoming more nurturing and involved in family care. We often hear the phrase, "He is a man of the nineties." What does that mean? Are men becoming more open, more expressive, more connected, more involved in family life? And if so, what impact do these changes have on older men and middle-aged men caring for elderly family members with severe memory loss? Today's male caregivers were socialized in an era with different gender expectations.

What impact do the present demographic trends of a growing aging population, smaller family size, greater sibling mobility, more women entering the work force, and an increasing number of men remarrying have on men? Does it mean that more men will find themselves suddenly thrust into a caregiving role, caring for ill wives and aging parents? A brief overview of these changing gender and demographic patterns are presented below so the reader will better understand factors that may influence male caregivers.

The questioning and examining of gender roles came to the forefront in the 1970s. The women's movement of the 1970s made men aware that they too are harmed by rigid gender roles that limit them from developing to their full potential (O'Neil, 1982; Harrison, 1978). The men most at risk for adhering to the rigid, stereotypic roles are the men who are caregiving now: middle-aged sons and, even more so, elderly husbands. These men were socialized under the "masculine mystique," which included some potentially deleterious values. The key elements of this mystique are as follows: control of self, others, and the environment are essential to proving one's masculinity; the expression of feelings and emotions should be avoided; seeking help and support is a sign of weakness; avoiding a display of vulnerability and intimacy with other men is imperative; a career is the measure of one's success (O'Neil, 1982).

This was what the male caregivers of today learned as they were growing up, especially older men. And as researchers have documented, the older men have learned it well. Recent studies have found that, in general, older men have fewer friends and no confidants after the death of a spouse; they are more self-reliant, rather than asking for help; they tend to suppress their feelings; they have more difficulty with retirement because of loss of work roles; and they tend to use mastery and control for coping strategies, often in situations where they may have little control (Dulac and Kosberg, 1994; Solomon, 1982; Barer, 1994). All these characteristics can have negative implications for elderly male caregivers. Some research

has shown that middle-aged sons have many of the same characteristics as these older men (Allen, 1994).

Feminist theorists have also proposed ways in which men have
been influenced by these rigid gender roles, which can also have an
impact on male caregiving. Carol Gilligan (1982) proposed that
because of these rigid roles, when faced with a moral dilemma (such
as caring for an ill family member), men act out of an ethic of duty,
while women act out of an ethic of caring. Thus, if extended to
caregiving, male caregivers would have less emotional involvement.
Ruddick (1989), in the same vein, suggests that as children, women
learn to connect and fuse with others, while men learn early on to
separate. It is this, perhaps, that impedes men from developing im
portant caregiving skills, such as establishing confidants and support networks.

Social science theorists, though, have hypothesized that as men
and women age, they may become more androgynous, lessening
rigid gender roles. Thus men would become more nurturing and
caring as they age. The movement toward androgyny for older men
would mean they would feel freer to take on new caregiving roles
and could allow themselves to enjoy and find much satisfaction
and meaning in this new role. There is some evidence that supports this premise of a movement toward androgyny as we age, but
much more research needs to be done (Bem, 1976; O'Neil, 1982;
Boles and Tatro, 1982).

As changing gender roles may influence the male caregivers in
this study, so will the large demographic changes that are rapidly
occurring in the United States. The most significant population trends
that will affect them are the increased longevity of the elderly, higher
rates of remarriage for men, smaller family size, increased mobility
of grown children, and higher rates of women entering the work
force (Himes, 1992).

We are a graying society in the United States and worldwide,
and both men and women are living longer. The size of the population in the United States over the age of 65 is expected to grow from
about 25.7 million elderly in 1980 to about 52 million in the year
2020 (U.S. Bureau of the Census, 1989). So, there will be more
older people in our population with more older men available to
take on the caregiving role, as well as more older women who may

need that care, as the incidence of severe memory loss and disability increases with age.

Another demographic factor that adds to the availability of older men for caregiving is that a majority of men who become widowed or who divorce tend to remarry. This is true for younger men as well as older men. Older men are six times more likely to remarry than older women (Himes, 1992) and, as discussed earlier, spouses are the most reliable and consistent caregivers.

Declining family size, the increased mobility of grown children, and more women entering the labor force will all have an impact on which family members will assume the majority of the responsibility of caregiving for ill parents. The proportion of one-child families has been increasing, the number of two-child families has remained the same, and the number of large families has been dramatically decreasing in the United States (U.S. Bureau of the Census, 1989). This factor, coupled with the increased mobility of grown children as they move across the country for employment, may make a man the most available person to provide care to an ill wife or parent. Also add to these demographic changes the participation of women in the labor market, which has increased dramatically over the last half-century. By the year 2000, over 50 percent of the women most likely to provide the care to impaired parents will be in the work force (Brody, 1990). All these demographic changes are destined to have an impact on men in our society.

Returning to our study on male caregivers, we have a group of 60 men, sons and husbands, whose gender socialization occurred under one set of "rules," and who are now providing care to impaired elderly family members in a changing time. Thus, we must ask the question proposed at the beginning of this section again: What impact do these slowly changing gender roles and demographic patterns have on male caregiving? A clear answer is not yet available. Some researchers say there has been little effect on the number of males now involved in caregiving tasks (Coverman and Sheley, 1986; Allen, 1994); other researchers disagree and believe that more elderly men will become involved in these tasks (Kaye and Applegate, 1994). More research on men in the caregiving role is needed, for either by choice or by default, increasing numbers of men will become the new caregivers of the 1990s and beyond.

Theoretical Frameworks

There are a number of theoretical frameworks that have been used to examine the impact on the families who care for elderly relatives; these frameworks can also be applied to male caregivers. The most often used and most well known is the stress and coping paradigm. The theory proposes that different levels of stressors and resources influence caregiver outcomes. Stresses for the caregiver refer to patient- and illness- related factors. Resources available to the caregivers include personal disposition, as well as social, environmental, and financial resources. The interactions of the different levels of these stressors and resources can have an impact on a caregiver's physical and emotional health in stressful situations (Pearlin and Schooler, 1978, Pearlin et al., 1990).

This framework provides much useful information about the caregiving experience. It gives us knowledge about the stresses, coping strategies, and resources of caregivers, as well as their impact on these people. For this study, we have included two general research questions derived from this framework: (1) What is it like for a man to take on a major caregiving role? and (2) How does a man adapt to and cope with his new functions?

Our goal in this book, though, is to provide a broad perspective and portray a larger picture of the experience of male caregivers than the stress and coping paradigm permits. For this broader perspective, we have also turned to a framework that focuses on the meaning a man finds in this caregiving experience and the motivations he has for taking on this uncharacteristic role. It is a combination of an existential paradigm that looks at how a person can grow and find meaning through experiencing a very difficult situation (Frankel, 1963, 1978; Farran et al., 1991) and the motivational/moral question of "Why care?" This question of why people take on these caregiving roles for the elderly is just beginning to be examined in the caregiving literature (McFadden, 1994; Schulz, 1990). From this framework two research questions were also included: (1) What are a man's motivations for taking on a caregiving role? and (2) What meaning does he derive from this caregiving experience?

The Study

This study is a collection of the narratives of 30 husbands and 30 sons caring for a spouse or parent with memory loss. These are stories of their experiences told to us through in-depth interviews. They are personal accounts of their caregiving and how this experience has affected their lives, not historically documented accounts (see Bertaux, 1981).

Because so little is known about the day-to-day experiences of men in a caregiving role, we chose a qualitative research approach. This approach allows us to examine closely the caregiving experiences of a small group of men in order to gain insights into the issues and concerns they face on a daily basis. This in-depth method of research also aids us in identifying commonalities and differences among male caregivers. Findings from such research can identify, for larger caregiver studies, issues that need to be further evaluated.

The focus of this caregiving study is on men only: husbands and sons. No comparisons are made to women caregivers. This way the men's voices will be heard unobstructed by gender comparisons. The information for this study was gathered in three stages from 1991 to 1994. The research originally started as a pilot study of 15 husbands caring for a wife with dementia. The sample was limited to men who were caring for their wives at home or who had in the last year placed their wives in a nursing home. Attempts were made in the sample to include husbands who depicted a broad range of relevant demographic factors such as socioeconomic class, race, urban/rural settings, number of years of caregiving, stage of the illness (early, middle, late), working/retired status, and support service usage.

At the end of the data collection and analysis, we discovered three major holes in the sample selection: Only one of the caregivers in the sample was African-American; husbands caring for wives who developed early onset dementia (dementia under the age of 60) were not part of the sample; and few men other than middle and upper middle class were included. To correct these gaps and to expand the sample size, we decided to do a second stage of data collection, and interviewed 15 more husbands. The broadening of the sample base was not done with the intent of it becoming a representative sample, because this is not the goal of qualitative research. Rather, it was done so this nonrandom sample would ensure the inclusion of a broad range of different types of husband caregivers, especially those not reached by the original sample selection.

The sample of husband caregivers for the study were all men who had contact with the local Alzheimer's Association chapter. The sample ranged from men who had called the association's helpline once, or received the bimonthly newsletter, or came to an educational workshop, or were part of a computer network, to men who attended a support group on a regular basis. One caregiver was an Alzheimer's Association board member. Advertisements were placed in the association newsletter and on the local Alzheimer's Association computer bulletin board. Alzheimer's Association staff members approached a few support group members whom they thought would be interested in the study and whose participation would broaden the demographic base. Helpline calls were screened for husband callers for two three-month periods by the Alzheimer's Association staff. A letter was then sent out by the association that explained the study and solicited participation. Staff actively recruited African-American participants. Following the research protocol of the association, in order to protect the privacy of their constituents, we were not directly given names of possible participants. An interested husband needed to initiate the phone call to us.

The third stage of the data collection was the recruitment of sons. After presenting the preliminary findings of the husbands study to a group at an Alzheimer's Association meeting, a son approached the first author (P.B.H.) to further discuss the results. He believed that the issues of son caregivers were always left out of studies, and that they had special needs, different from other caregivers. He felt it was time they "were listened to." After discussing his concerns and speaking with other sons, a third stage of the study was initiated.

Because fewer sons are involved in caring for an elderly parent with dementia, the sons sample had fewer restrictions placed on it. The sample included not only sons who took on the major caregiving role for their parents but also those who were not main caregivers but who were actively involved in their parents' care. In this second group of sons, the other parent was still alive and living with his/her demented spouse as the major caregiver. Our main focus was, as in the husbands research, on sons caring for a parent at home; however, sons who were still caring for a parent who had moved to a nursing home were included as well. Also included were sons who had cared for a parent at home who had died within the last five years. As in the husbands sample, we tried to include a broad range of son caregivers, including African-American and white sons, sons from various socioeconomic classes, and sons caring for a parent in the various stages of dementia. Not included were sons who were long-distance caregivers, although there were sons in this category who were interested in participating in the study.

The 30 sons for the study were recruited in a similar manner as the husbands, but with two differences: A larger number of sons responded to the ads in the newsletter than husbands, and sons were less likely to have been recruited through a support group. Again active recruitment was necessary to obtain African-American sons as participants.

The Interviews

The majority of the interviews were conducted (28 husbands and 30 sons) by the first author (P.B.H.). Another husband interview was conducted by one of her students, who had accompanied her on a number of the other interviews. One husband interview was conducted by the other author (J.B.).

The interviews were onetime interviews that lasted approximately from one to two-and-a-half hours. The interviews of husbands tended to be longer and most often took place in their homes. The interviews of sons were shorter and most often took place in their offices, the researcher's office, or at a restaurant.

For both sons and husbands, an interview guide approach was used. We developed a set of topics, one for husbands and one for sons, to cover in the course of the interview (see Appendix A for interview guides). The topics or major issues to be explored by the guides were derived from the research questions and selected from the caregiving literature and from discussions with health care professionals. The topics were pretested in interviews with four male caregivers, two husbands and two sons, who were not included in this study. With this interview guide approach, interviews were run as conversations with the topics weaved into the conversations as the flow permitted. The exact wording varied from conversation to conversation.

The interviews always started out in the same way. The purpose of the study was explained, and the caregiver was told the interview would be conducted like a conversation with specific topics woven into it. It was then suggested that the interviewee begin by telling a little bit about his wife's or parent's situation, and to start at a place that made most sense to him. Usually this prompting opened an outpouring of thoughts and emotions, and there were very few pauses in the flow. Occasionally the interview was difficult; some men had trouble expressing themselves. In these instances, we followed the interview guide fairly closely. More structure seemed to help those particular men.

We were often amazed at how willing these men, both husbands and sons, were to tell their caregiving stories and share their experiences with a complete stranger. For many of these men, this interview was a therapeutic experience, and they often said they felt better at the end of the interview. One son, immediately after the interview, called the director of the local Alzheimer's Association and told her, "I am not sure I helped the study, but boy, was it therapeutic for me." Another son, whose father died a few weeks after the interview, wrote a note of thanks to the researcher for giving him and his brother the opportunity to talk about their father. This son said the experience made it much easier for them to come to terms with their father's death. In these interviews, as suggested by Fontana and Frey (1994) and Oakley (1981), real conversation took place and often an empathetic understanding was reached.

The time and place of the interviews were arranged at the convenience of the men. Most husbands, as they were still living with and caring for their wives, met with us in the kitchen or living room of their homes. Occasionally the wives were present and participated in the interview, depending on the level of the wife's impairment and the state of the marital relationship. This decision was left up to the discretion of the husband. If a wife was not present during the interview, she was often introduced to us at the end of the session.

The sons, on the other hand, preferred and were able to meet in more neutral places, such as their offices or in the university office of the researcher (P.B.H.). On two occasions, sons were met at local restaurants, and an interview with one son took place in a public library. Sons preferred not to be interviewed at home, and only two sons included their wives in the interview.

All the interviews were taped, with the men's permission; no one refused. The tapes were then transcribed and reviewed against the field notes completed after each interview. The analysis consisted of a six-step procedure, four of which the authors did separately. First, we read the entire transcription of an interview. Then we re-read the transcript for a second time to develop substantive codes for each narrative. In other words, for each interview, we looked for the repetition of certain words, phrases, or meanings that explained the caregiving experience for each man, an approach suggested by Glaser and Strauss (1967). Third, we grouped these codes into themes that emerged out of these codes, such as commitment, social isolation, and love. We developed a master list of themes from each interview that would allow for easy cross-interview examination. Fourth, we looked for quotations that summarized the essence of each man's experience as a caregiver. In searching for meaningful quotations, we posed the following questions to ourselves: What was the caregiving experience like for him? and What did it mean to him? In the fifth stage of the analysis, we compared our findings. In areas of disagreement, those portions of the transcripts were re-read and discussed until we reached agreement. The final step was a content analysis of the taped interviews using features of the WordPerfect software program. The computerized content analysis was then compared with our other analyses for consistencies and differences.

In the following chapters, names have been changed for privacy and confidentiality. The excerpts of the interviews have not been changed, and reflect the expressions and statements of the sons and husbands who participated in the study.

Before concluding this section, it is important to remind the reader that, as in most qualitative studies, the authors were not neutral spectators, with the bias that might entail. We participated in the conversations, and thus were collaborators in the development of these narratives. We have also selected which men's words to present to you and have developed the analytic framework from which to view this information. Thus, in truth, this research became a joint endeavor between the authors and the husbands and sons who participated in the study.

Part One

Husbands as Caregivers

Their Inner World

Chapter Two
Husbands' Characteristics, Common Themes, and Shared Experiences

The common denominator that linked these 30 husbands was their providing care for a wife with dementia. The predominant cause of this dementia was Alzheimer's disease, but some wives had related disorders. In a discussion with one of the first men we interviewed, three stages of dementia through which he saw his wife progress were described: an early, a middle, and a late stage. Because the other husbands in the study could relate well to this man's definition of the stages, we used them as a common basis in our discussions.

The early stage of dementia was described as including the symptoms of mild forgetfulness with some repetitive questioning and some occasional confusion about people and places. One of the husbands caring for a wife in this early stage described this experience well.

Sometimes she won't come to bed with me. She thinks I'm my brother. She says, "You ain't got no business going to bed with me." I've known her to sit up all night rather than go to bed with me. Now that gets me down a little, I'll be frank with you. He continued, turning to his wife who had just joined us, "And you ask the same questions over and over again. His wife replied, "Well, there is nobody here, but you and me, and if I have a question, who am I going to ask if I don't ask you?"

Another husband caring for his wife in the early stage described his experience:

There are differences in her behavior, especially in the kitchen. She can't remember where things are. She can't cook anymore. She's getting forgetful. I use lots of notes all over the house to remind her, the refrigerator, the bed stand, wherever's near.

Many husbands portrayed the middle stage as a period when their wives exhibited increased behavior problems, such as agitation, wandering, confusion, and increased forgetfulness. Her communication skills became impaired and she needed supervision of personal care and hygiene. Many of the husbands talked about their fear of their wives wandering away from the house during this stage of the disease. One husband related his experience with his wife.

You hear about the need for special locks or buzzers on the door and I tried not to do it. But for some reason all of a sudden she gets up in the middle of the night and says, "Well, I think I'll go home." I tried to convince her she was home, but when I went to the bathroom she ran out of the house. She moves very quietly and I looked around and I hollered and nobody answered. She was out and way up the street already.

Husbands described the last stage as a time when their wives were no longer able to speak or recognize family members. Their wives often needed complete personal care assistance and were often no longer mobile. Men caring for wives in this last stage of dementia often told us how they fed their wives, which sometimes took three hours, as well as how they dressed them, changed them, and put them to bed. One husband even sang to his wife and said her prayers for her, as he put her to sleep.

The 30 husbands came from various backgrounds and circumstances: age, education, occupation, religion, ethnicity, and economic situations. At this time in their lives, however, the experience of caring for a wife with dementia was the dominant factor that bridged these differences. As we interviewed these husbands, not only were they also very willing to share their experiences with us, they were very interested in learning how other men were dealing with similar situations.

Characteristics of the Husbands

The men in the study had a diverse demographic profile (see Appendix B, Table 1). The majority of the men lived either in Cleveland or the five-county area surrounding the city, a mixture of urban and rural settings. A few lived in apartments, but most lived in their own houses. Some homes were old, small four-room bungalows;

others were large modern homes, and some were town houses in retirement centers.

The ages of the husbands spanned five decades. The youngest man was 41 years old, a truck driver in the height of his career. The oldest man was 91 years old, a retired physician; he had finally retired for the third time at age 80.

Dementia, particularly the Alzheimer's type, knows no age bounds, but its incidence increases with age. This is indicated by the 72-year-old average age of the husbands and the 71-year-old average age of the wives with the disease. Alzheimer's disease also reaches across all ethnic and racial boundaries. The men in the sample were predominantly white, and 20 percent of the sample was African American, well above the 8 percent of elderly African Americans in the population nationally.

Most of the husbands had retired from their diverse jobs: factory workers, accountants, carpenters, teachers, custodians, small-business owners, construction workers, engineers, and business executives. Their incomes varied as well: 27 percent of the sample had incomes under $10,000, and 27 percent of the sample had incomes over $40,000 (see Appendix B, Table 1). Some men faced the difficult decision each month of determining which medications they would not buy so they could afford to eat. A few had just finished building special houses and additions designed to better meet the needs of their wives' failing health.

These men were in their marriages for the long haul (average 44.3 years), though a few were second marriages. During the interviews, we frequently spent time looking at family photo albums that often spanned half a century. Pictures of fiftieth wedding anniversaries hung on the walls. As one man reminded us, "Isn't that what the marriage license says? For better or for worse? There ain't no promiscuity, nothing like that in our generation. You don't get that today."

The average number of years a wife had been diagnosed with dementia was 5.6 years. Some men were new to the caregiving experience, involved for less than a year; others had a decade and a half of caregiving experience.

Many men hired people to help them with this care; 47 percent of the sample used respite care in the home. Others did it on their own. The majority of men in the sample, 60 percent, had children in town. Most of the children provided some kind of respite for their fathers, be it one night a week out, every weekend, or a few hours a month.

The most often-used services by these husband caregivers were support groups, with 60 percent of the sample participating (probably a reflection of how the sample was drawn). Many of the men whose wives were in the early stage of dementia attended a specialized support group designed for families and their diagnosed relative in the early stage. The Alzheimer's Association helpline (information & referral calls), educational programs, and educational literature were services often used by the husbands. Thirty percent of the sample utilized other services, including Alzheimer's assessment centers, computer bulletin boards on Alzheimer's disease (which will be explained in Chapter 4), and counseling services.

The husband caregivers in this sample indeed have some similar characteristics as well as much contrast among them. They represent not a random sample, but a broad range of caregivers.

Common Themes and Shared Experiences

Across the 30 husbands interviewed, 11 common themes related to their caregiving were revealed during the course of our conversations. The themes were a commitment to caregiving, the reactions to the medical diagnosis, the range of emotions, the feeling of social isolation, the losses, the significance of cooking, the types of coping strategies used, the role of children, a sense of purpose, a feeling of accomplishment, and a sense of hope. This section of the chapter will explore these themes. Taken together they give us clues about the inner world of men caring for wives with dementia.

Before starting this section, however, the reader should note that although we and other gerontologists refer to these men as "caregivers," this term is foreign to them. They did not define themselves by that term, nor did most of them know what it meant. The men viewed themselves foremost simply as husbands caring for ill wives. This is quite different from the cold approach implied by the terms "caregiver" and "care recipient" used by most researchers.

Commitment

The commitment of these men in caring for their wives was a dominant feature of the relationships described in the interviews. Their commitment was expressed in many different ways. A number of caregivers almost word-for-word said, "You don't understand; if it was me who was ill, she would do double what I am doing for her." Other men had their own unique way of discussing their feeling of commitment.

One 71-year-old African-American man caring for his wife in the early stages of Alzheimer's shared his thoughts about commitment:

This is a challenge. Can you be good now? Has she been good to you? I got a car outside. If three tires are going all right and one goes flat, you don't say the car should be dumped. Fix the tire. I've told her, "I've known you a lifetime almost, so I ain't goin' to jump ship now, honey"; it doesn't work that way.

An 80-year-old husband was providing care to his wife, who was moving into the middle stage of the disease. He stated, "I am dedicating my whole life to my wife; I don't resent it. My whole thoughts are for my wife." Another 84-year-old man whose wife was in the late stage of dementia commented, "You do what you have to do . . . you do your best for her. It seems like you're just trying to care for her until she wears out."

These 30 husband caregivers were committed to providing care for their ill wives. The men said it in diverse ways, but the meaning was clear.

Reactions to Medical Diagnosis

Almost unanimously the husbands complained about some issue concerning their wife's diagnosis: the length of time it took to make the diagnosis, the way they were treated by health care professionals, the lack of compassion some physicians showed for their situation. Over and over again this became an integral part of the interviews. Only one husband felt, as he put it, "part of the team."

The time of diagnosis is a very difficult emotional period for families and the individual with the dementing illness (Haley, Clair, and Saulsberry, 1992). As one husband succinctly put it,

*The day the Doc gave me the diagnosis—I'll tell you it hit me with 20
tons of bricks. I just . . . had so many questions. The first, and I think
maybe the obvious question, how long? How much time do I have left
with her? I didn't have the guts. I didn't have the energy. I knew I couldn't
control my emotions enough to ask him anything. I just said, "Thanks,
Doc, good-bye."*

Many of the husbands told us that it would have helped them immensely during this initial diagnosis period to be told directly that
their wife had Alzheimer's disease. They often left the offices of the
doctors and hospitals uncertain of what the diagnosis was. (In all
fairness, it is a difficult disease to diagnose.) The men felt that if they
better understood their wife's condition, they could have dealt with
it more realistically. They believed it is possible to give a clear diagnosis without taking away hope. At one point in an interview, one
of the husbands stated his feelings:

*No one ever comes right out directly and says Alzheimer's, but we ran
test after test after test trying to find the problem. They all say memory
loss, dementia. But they gave us a number of pamphlets to read that said
Alzheimer's. So from that point on, we realized what was happening.*

As evidenced from the quotations above, this initial diagnosis period was a critical time for the husbands we interviewed. It was an
unsolicited topic that came up again and again.

Range of Emotions
The men in our interviews expressed a full range of emotions about
their situation. The most common ones were anger frustration, pain,
and despondency. Yet, in spite of all these negative feelings, many
men were still able to feel compassion for their wives.

Anger and frustration were the most common emotions expressed. One 91-year-old man whose wife was in the middle stage of
the disease responded, "There are times she won't cooperate. I sometimes get angry and yell at her. It hurts me. Oh, it hurts her. She
hates when I start yelling. I can't control myself."

Another man, 61 years old, whose wife was in early onset dementia, admitted, "There are many things that she did that totally

infuriated me. I would throw plates, just smash them against the wall. I smoke a pipe and I bet I broke ten pipes, just totally smashed them."

Another 91-year-old, whose his was wife in the early stage, acknowledged his anger also:

I cannot accept the change in her. I know, of course, it is the disease, but I don't want to accept the fact. It makes me mad. I tell her, "What the hell are you doing that for?" This is crazy and I will react in that manner until I've had a little time to adjust, and it doesn't happen in a minute and it doesn't happen in an hour. It takes a while. Then after the time goes by, then I can accept it, and then something else pops up and I react in the same way. It's just absolutely unreasonable and I know it.

This intensity of anger is not felt by all the men, but different levels of anger and frustration were evident in many of the interviews. Despondency and despair were also present. Some men had worked through these feelings, and others at the time of the interview had not.

This despair was best described by a 61-year-old husband. He shared with us one of his journal entries: "Sometimes I feel like Joe Pfssst . . . the character from Dick Tracy who always had a dark cloud and flies around him."

An 80-year-old man disclosed, "It's not very nice when you see you lose part of your wife . . every day a little piece. We had a good marriage." He continued: "I really get down in the dumps. It hit me, hit me so damn hard."

Yet, even in the midst of such despair and anger, many men are able to feel compassion and empathy for their wives. The 80-year-old husband went on to say the following about his wife:

It's very difficult for her; everyone's feeling sorry for the caregiver. She is the one who really needs the help. I don't need it. She could cook, make dresses for the kids, make herself a coat and hat. She lost all that. Sometimes she gets very sentimental and blue. She feels bad, shaking and sobbing. She sometimes wakes up to the fact that I am her husband and she can't even remember her own husband.

These male caregivers experienced a range of emotions, some positive and some negative, as they provided support and care to their wives in varying stages of dementia. Husbands whose wives were in the early and middle stages of dementia expressed more anger, frustration, and despair than men whose wives were in the last stage. These men had worked through the negative feelings and could voice a sense of accomplishment (discussed below).

The negative impact of caregiving has been labeled by researchers as "caregiver burden and stress," but none of the husbands ever used that phrase in talking with us. The emotions these men expressed go much deeper than the terms "caregiver burden" or "stress" connote.

Social Isolation

Social isolation from family, especially from friends, was a very common theme. Friends stopped coming to visit because they were uncomfortable seeing the woman's deterioration and because they didn't know what to say. A 75-year-old man, caring for a wife in the middle stage of dementia, poignantly mentioned: "Most of the couples we were friendly with, we originally met through my wife. I felt funny calling them up after she became ill." He added, "Strangers are more of a help than your real friends; they don't come by anymore."

A 76-year-old caregiver who had just placed his wife in a nursing home told us: "My minister would come by once a month and we would go out to lunch. I would look forward to that one constant human contact." And yet another caregiver, a 64-year-old man whose wife had early onset dementia, diagnosed nine years earlier when she was 53, related his disappointment in friends and family.

People don't come around any more. They stay away. It used to bother me. It doesn't anymore. Some people you thought very highly of, you never see anymore. Some people you only saw occasionally come out of the woodwork now. This not only happens to friends, it happens within the family. So your whole outlook on things changes.

For many of these men, their wives were their main link to the social world of friends. As their wives' dementia progressed, friends felt uncomfortable and pulled away, and the men, who depended upon their wives' social skills to connect them to others, felt doubly isolated.

Losses

These men experienced multiple losses. The most common losses the men expressed to us were loss of a companion and confidant, loss of meaningful sexual intimacy, loss of one's former identity, loss of control, and loss of future plans and dreams.

The loss of female companionship added to the feelings of social isolation. One 68-year-old husband, who had been caring for his wife for 10 years, stated, "Women look at things differently; I'm not talking about sex now, but I miss having a conversation with women. I found that whenever I go to the grocery store, I try to strike up casual conversations with the female shoppers and the checkout clerks."

Loss of sexual intimacy with their wives was a topic very difficult for many of the men to discuss. Turning off the tape recorder during this section of the interview often helped in facilitating the discussion of this topic. The sexual aspect of their relationship had lost its meaning, and for many husbands this lessened their sexual interest in their wives. They were struggling to come to terms with the conflict between their normal sex drive and their loyalty to their wives.

Some of the men were interested in discussing with us how other husbands we had interviewed were handling this issue. One husband divulged on tape that "the change in the sexual relationship with your wife is a difficult thing to go through, most especially for someone who is younger. You wonder, 'How should I behave?'"

A 64-year-old caregiver poignantly voiced another loss alluded to by other caregivers, a loss of sense of identity (how one defines who one is), in this man's case, his sense of manliness.

After being in this [caregiving] for awhile, you begin to lose your male identity. A woman is used to everything in the house, so the role comes as probably a routine. Now you reverse the situation and a man has to learn all this. Now where does he go for the answers? It's very confusing. You're going to have to do some cooking, cleaning, washing, dusting, spots on clothes, this, that. It is a whole new learning process. I've been in construction all my life. To go from that to this was quite a transition, yes. Your whole psychological outlook on things changes. You don't view things as you did before. You begin to question who you are.

Loss of control in their lives was another dominant theme for a majority of these men. Alzheimer's disease had brought disorder, confusion, and unpredictability into their lives and homes. A 61-year-old husband caring for his 54-year-old wife with early onset dementia revealed his loss of control:

I realized my life was changed forever. After the first MRI, I'm not sure of the exact moment, I began the first day of the rest of my life. I would never again be able to have a job in the traditional way, the job being away from the home. I knew my wife needed somebody in attendance to oversee her.

He continued,

The most difficult thing for me is self-control. I go into what I refer to as uncontrollable rage and this is the woman I love. So many things are out of my control and I haven't totally learned to realize that. Damnit, I'm tired.

The loss of dreams and plans for the future together was another common theme of these husbands. The loss of dreams about traveling together in their retirement years and the loss of sharing together the joys of grandparenthood were the two most often mentioned lost dreams. Some of the wives with early onset dementia never knew those grandchildren who were born after their descent into the latter stages of the disease. So their husbands faced grandparenthood alone.

Many of the men had hoped to travel to Europe or across the United States with their wives and now were unable to do so. One 74-year-old husband, caring for a wife in the middle stage of dementia, said wistfully about his plans:

In '91 we went to the Maritime Provinces in Canada. That was really one of the nicest trips of our career. It was like time rolled back 15 years. It was a wonderful trip. But I don't know when we will try that again. And with some of the other problems that have come up recently . . . even going in the car, trips are getting shorter and shorter.

As voiced by these husbands, the losses for many of these men were on various levels and in numerous areas of their lives. But a sense of utter despair and hopelessness was not the impression that we were left with at the conclusion of the interviews. A sense of hope was still evident for most men, as will be discussed later in this chapter.

The Significance of Cooking

Cooking took on a special significance for these husbands. Of all the new tasks and skills they needed to learn, almost unanimously, cooking was mentioned as the task they disliked the most. This was true also for the few husbands who already had cooking skills before their wives' illness. Cooking, to these men, symbolized much more than the actual chore of preparing a meal; it had multiple meanings.

On one level it reminded the men of the loss of their wives and companions. Most of the husbands were proud of their wives' cooking abilities prior to the onset of the dementia. They also mentioned that cooking was one of the first household activities the woman could no longer do. For these men, part of their wife's identity was that she was a good cook; the loss of that function was for them the loss of a part of their wife, herself.

One 91-year-old husband, reminiscing about his wife's cooking, remarked, "My wife used to be a very high-class cook. She used to bake the most delicious cakes and cookies. People when they passed the house could smell them." Another husband stated, "She was such a wonderful cook, and that's the first thing she lost was cooking. Her career was a housewife, and the first thing she lost was her knack for cooking. Now she has to depend on me, and I'm the worst."

On another level, cooking, or food, in our society takes on social meaning. We use food to establish and maintain social relationships among family as well as friends. These men often talked about the social activities surrounding food that they used to enjoy with their wives: going out to dinner, or conversations in the kitchen or over the dining room table at the evening meal. The need to take on the chore of cooking also increased these men's feelings of social isolation.

Another husband, 68 years old, caring for his wife in the middle stage of dementia, when asked what had been the most stressful part of caregiving for him, responded, "Cooking! I bought one of those

Chinese woks. Boy, was it great for about a week. Then I got tired of it, chopping up all those vegetables and doing it by myself."

On a more basic level, food is used to nourish the ones we love and care about. It is often used to demonstrate our love, and in some ethnic cultures it is equated with love. Thus it is not surprising that, when asked which activity has been the most difficult to take on, cooking was the response the men most often gave.

Coping Strategies

There were a number of common coping strategies these caregivers used: maintaining control, using a problem-solving approach, arranging respite care, establishing a structured regime, allowing time for themselves outside of the home, and relying on strong religious beliefs.

Maintaining control over their caregiving was a crucial issue for these husbands. It was a strategy that allowed them to cope with a situation in which they felt helpless over the process of the disease and the devastation it wrought on their wives. Many men echoed the belief that "no one takes better care of her than I do," and they were reluctant to give up any part of that care. As one 91-year-old husband caring for a wife in the early stage stated, "Men are used to being in charge and they are not used to being wrong or not knowing what to do."

Comments by another 91-year-old man with a wife in the middle stage of dementia illustrated this concept well:

I cook her breakfast. I make her bed. I clean the house, wash the dishes, take care of everything. The aides [who come to help] are good with their attention, but there's nothing like flesh and blood. I can dress and undress her faster than anybody else.

This control was often coupled with a problem-solving approach. It was best exemplified by one 78-year-old husband who said: "I am a doer; I see what needs to be done and I do it." A 77-year-old husband caring for a wife in the last stage of Alzheimer's demonstrated this problem-solving approach.

I wish somehow or other that the knowledge over the years had been available in capsule form in the beginning. It is, to a degree, if you know what to read. But there are the little things that you have to do, at least I do, just kind of lumber along until I finally stumble on the answers. I presume what works for one doesn't work on another patient in many cases. It's been an interesting, challenging situation.

The use of respite care, whether in-home care, day care, or vacation care, was a major coping strategy of the men who had been caring for their wives for many years. Men in the early stages of caregiving, who were more often in a crisis stage, had not yet built into their routine some sort of respite care, but were strongly considering it. As one 68-year-old husband caring for a wife in the later stage of Alzheimer's said, "It's those times away that keep me sane; then I'm ready to come back and take care of my wife again." The 77-year-old husband mentioned in the quotation above echoed almost those exact words. The first thing he said in the interview was, "You have to have a physical separation between the wives and their husbands during the day. Every book I've read tells you the same thing. It is imperative."

The majority of male caregivers used respite care to do things outside of their home for their own enjoyment. This usually involved some outdoor recreational activity, ranging from golfing, walking, and bike riding to ballroom dancing and motorcycle riding. They needed to feel that they still had a life. For some men, participating in activities that they used to do meant a continuation of or a link to their former lives. One 64-year-old husband, whose wife has early onset dementia, shared the following with us:

I keep busy. I play golf. Occasionally there will be tournaments and outings and I'll play in them. I do projects around the house, but I really have no business even starting new projects. But I do them because for me that is like putting me back to where I was before. It helps me regroup and become a little stronger.

It seemed that the men who had been caring for their wives for the longest period of time expressed the least burden and the most satisfaction with their arrangements. They were able to work out a routine that was acceptable to them. A phrase often used by these

husband caregivers was "setting up a system that works." For each
man, that system varied depending upon the wives' condition and
their economic situation. Most men arose at a certain time every
day and followed a prescribed routine. Some men had paid help that
assisted in their wives' care and provided them respite. Other men
had family members—children, siblings, cousins—who would come
routinely, perhaps once a week, and provide some assistance. It was
this "system" that effectively allowed them to deal with their wives'
dementia.

A final coping strategy that helped many of the husbands deal
with the difficult situations they faced with their wives in the downward spiral of a devastating illness was their spirituality, their religion, and their faith in God. This faith went across denominations.
For some men it meant regular church attendance or active participation in church activities. For other men it was more a personal/
spiritual relationship with God. Whatever form it took, it provided
many men with comfort.

As one 61-year-old man said, "Religion has had a vital role in my
education. From a religious point of view, it has brought us much closer
to God during this whole thing. I have always had a personal relationship with God . . . I told him, just don't hit me so fast with things."

One 74-year-old African-American husband discussed with us
his faith in God.

*God in time will take care of a lot of things. We have to change and
condition ourselves to accept it. I accept what the Bible says. I try to live
with it. It's my business to know if this is His will, I must adjust. You
pray and you pray and you pray. The priority is humanity and believing
in Him, knowing that in time He will take care of it.*

Role of Children
The role children should play in this caregiving process was also
commonly discussed. Most of the husbands caring for their wives
had very few expectations and made limited demands on their children, be they daughters or sons. These husbands said almost word
for word, "My wife is my problem. Our children have lives of their
own. I don't expect them to do much for me. They help out when I
need some time off."

A few husbands were disappointed by the lack of attention the children showed their mothers. Some husbands accepted it and felt their children could not deal with their mother's illness. Other husbands were very angry with their children. As one 80-year-old husband said, "My son lives on the west side of town [across town from his parents], and I talk and talk to him that he should see his mother more, and he feels and he cries, but the minute he's away it's all forgotten."

A few of the husbands became closer to their children because of their wives' illness. One 90-year-old husband spoke of how his daughter, who lives near by, had become his confidant, and of the pleasure this closeness has brought to him.

In our discussions with the 30 husbands caring for their wives with dementia and the difficulties, pain, and stresses they experienced, it would be easy to overlook the positive experiences of these men. But, as the interviews revealed, there are positive aspects associated with the experience of caregiving. There were three areas in particular to which the men alluded: the sense of purpose or meaning caregiving brought to their lives, a sense of accomplishment or personal growth, and a sense of hope.

Meaning and a Sense of Purpose

One 68-year-old caregiver, who had been caring for his wife for 10 years, said, "My wife's illness is a mixed blessing; it in a sense gives me a purpose around which to organize my activities. I am enjoying my retirement. It's not what we had planned, but it's not as awful as people think." An 80–year-old caregiver whose wife is in the middle stage of dementia stated purposefully, "I'm dedicating my life to my wife."

One 74-year-old caregiver with a wife in the early stage of Alzheimer's disease took another approach. He shared with us, "This may be a challenge for me [from God]. Are you a good husband or not? Other people have been tested. Job was tested. So who am I? I'll get stronger! Adversity makes you stronger if you take it in a positive manner."

Sense of Accomplishment

The husband caregivers were often surprised at their accomplishments, their ability to take on a caregiver role that was foreign to them. This was most often true for the long-term caregiver, whose wife was in the last stage of dementia. One 76-year-old man who had been caring for his wife for 15 years stated, "Who would have thought I could do all this?"

A number of other men talked about the caregiving experience as being a personal growth process. This theme was expressed by one 68-year-old husband who stated, "I've found this experience with my wife, as difficult as it has been, has made me a better person. I've become more compassionate, more thoughtful. Twenty years ago, I could never have visualized myself doing this."

Another husband who had been caring for his wife with Alzheimer's for 12 years remarked about his experience.

Well, it makes you stronger. It makes you a better person, really. I always said if I didn't have my wife, I'd probably be a drunk or something like that. It gives you a little more quality to your life. I don't know, maybe it extends your life a little longer. It very much gives your life purpose. It gives you something to strive for and do.

Hope

The majority of men had not given up hope, hope that a cure would be found, hope for a better life, and just hope in general. As one 77-year-old husband said, "I wish we could somehow or another get the message out that you don't have to give up if you have Alzheimer's. There are lots of activities you can do. You don't have to become isolated." Another 80-year-old husband remarked, "When there is no hope, there is nothing left, is there? I keep hoping that they'll come up with a pill to eliminate Alzheimer's. If you remember the Salk pill, it eliminated polio. I haven't given up."

So even through the ordeal of caring for a wife with dementia, optimistic, hopeful, and affirming attitudes were still present in many of the men we encountered.

Conclusion

Over the course of our interviews with 30 husbands caring for a wife with dementia, 11 themes were constantly present: Commitment, medical diagnosis, range of emotions, social isolation, loss, cooking, coping strategies, role of children, and a sense of purpose, accomplishment, and hope were the motifs that appeared again and again in our conversations. This in-depth portrayal of the inner experiences of husband caregivers sheds new light on the male caregiving experience, different than many of the previous studies depicted.

These husbands were intensely and emotionally involved in caring for their wives, providing hands-on care for long periods of time. They did not necessarily seek outside assistance to help provide the care. They used respite as time for themselves, to keep their spirits up so they could continue caring for their wives.

The men did use a problem-solving approach, and they tried to set up systems that worked for them. Control was a critical issue, one that they tried to maintain. In fact, the majority of these men were struggling to blend dichotomous parts of themselves together: the rational and the emotional, instrumental and affective, the male and the female. For many, a movement toward androgyny was in progress.

Chapter Three
Toward a Typology of Husband Caregivers

The 30 men we interviewed had much in common, yet from these interviews, major patterns of divergence surfaced. There emerged five different types of male caregivers or different ways husbands oriented or adjusted themselves to their new caregiving role. The types reflect the major themes discussed in the previous chapter, but they also have characteristics and behavior patterns that are unique unto themselves.

Each group or type acclimated to their new caregiver role differently and experienced their situation differently. These five categories are "the worker," "labor of love," "sense of duty," "going it together," and "men in transition." Narratives of fourteen husbands' experiences with caregiving will be presented as a way of illustrating the differences among these five groups of men caring for a wife with dementia.

"The Worker"

This group of male caregivers adjusted to the new caregiver role by modeling their behavior after their world of work. Caregiving became a new work identity for them. Instead of being a salesman or an accountant, each was now a "caregiver." These men had set up mini-offices in their houses with desks, phones, and sometimes computers, and were handling their caregiving duties as a new work role. Each morning they would get up and schedule their days as though they were at the office. This was a role that was comfortable and familiar to them, and allowed them to adapt their skills to a new task.

Mr. Hansen

We first met Mr. Hansen three years ago; he was one of the first men we interviewed for this study. Over the past few years our paths have

crossed many times, as we found ourselves on a number of committees together working on issues related to Alzheimer's disease. Our
initial impressions of Mr. Hansen and his orientation toward his
caregiving role have been reinforced by these contacts.

When we first interviewed Mr. Hansen, he was an active, 76-
year-old white retired army officer who approached life with a sense
of humor and a pragmatic philosophy. Even though he is now dealing with a critical illness himself, his outlook and view on life has
not changed. He is a planner, and his initial words to us still direct
his life today, as he cares for his wife, who is in the early stage of
dementia. He imparted his motto to us, "I live by the six P's: Prior
Planning Prevents Piss-Poor Performance."

Mr. Hansen and his wife of 50 years live in a comfortable house
in a middle-class suburb. While reminiscing about their life together,
Mr. Hansen commented about his situation:

*We had a lot of fun together. I don't know what else to say except that we
enjoy life. Sure it bothers me to know she is affected this way, but it doesn't
change my feelings in any shape or form. I've been shot at [referring to his
wife's diagnosis], but I didn't get hit. It didn't severely ruin my lifestyle.*

Mrs. Hansen still enjoys the women's bowling league of which she is
a long-standing member. With some supervision she bowls a good
game, although when she returns home she cannot remember bowling that morning. Mrs. Hansen can perform light household tasks,
with supervision. Although her social skills are still intact, she is
quite repetitive in her conversation.

In order to get through the days, Mr. Hansen refers back to his
motto:

*You have to have a schedule. I have taken to planning our meals a week
in advance. I've been writing menus ahead—breakfast, lunch, supper—
and lay it out so there is something she can see. We stick to the same
schedule, same routine, up at 6:30 A.M. and to bed at 9:00 P.M. I'm
doing more planning than I have ever done in my entire life.*

His wife's main problem at the moment is short-term memory loss.
He compares his wife's difficulty to a computer that is having trouble

retrieving stored information. He has dealt with this problem by becoming her "RAM." He has had his wife assessed, and she is participating as a research subject in a clinical Alzheimer's disease drug trial at a local university hospital research center.

Mr. Hansen has an office with a computer set up in a spare bedroom of the house, where he organizes his wife's health care information and medical appointments. He spends many hours on the computer each week updating his records and using the modem to get the most up-to-date information on Alzheimer's disease. He has become an active member of a computer resource and support center for Alzheimer's caregivers.

Mr. Hansen ended the interview with some advice for other male caregivers. He stated, "I suggest they try to be as flexible as possible. You need to think of all your experiences, and then try and cast them into a new role; acquire new skills and build new patterns."

Mr. Gimmel

Mr. Gimmel is a very articulate, 78-year-old white male who approaches life, as he says, "with a sense of humor and good common sense." He greeted us at the door of his cramped one-bedroom apartment with a chef's hat on; he had just finished cooking a pot of chicken soup. The odor of the soup permeated the entire floor of the apartment building on one of the hottest days of the year. He proudly assured us, after we politely declined his invitation to have a bowl, that his soup was not any of that "canned store variety."

Mr. Gimmel never completed college and describes himself as a self-made man who reads everything. He had various careers from delivery van driver to small-business owner. He takes much delight in fighting the bureaucracy, particularly the medical bureaucracy. He has serious heart problems, and he is feisty and committed to caring for his wife. He worries much about what will happen to her if he can no longer care for her. As he says, "I watch her like a hawk. It's the least I can do. She took darn good care of me for fifty-four years."

Mrs. Gimmel is 75 years old and is in the early stage of Alzheimer's disease. She is very pleasant and socially appropriate, although she does acknowledge that her memory is failing. Mr.

Gimmel complained about her periods of mild confusion, at times not recognizing him. Their one daughter lives out of town, and contact with her is mostly by phone. She is their major shopper for nonfood items. Mr. Gimmel does the research, reading what brand is the best for their money. He then calls his daughter, who goes to a large discount store in New York and buys and ships the item to them.

He is the sole caregiver of his wife, receiving no outside services. As he stated, "They [paid help] won't be as conscientious as I." He has organized one part of their living room as his office, and each morning he sits down and plans out his work schedule for helping his wife.

I'm the laundress, cook, shopper, podiatrist. I keep my phone right here on my desk, and battle daily with Medicare and Blue Cross to make sure they follow up. I can hold my own. I also read everything I can about Alzheimer's and clip and save it in this box.

When asked how he learned to care for his wife, he explained his methods.

I read an awful lot. And I watched how my wife took care of her mother, with the little separate dishes for pills, and I incorporated that into my schedule.

Most of the conversation with Mr. Gimmel centered around the tasks he performs for his wife, including her daily walks, having her exercise to improve her gait, and installing grab bars in the bathroom. When asked for advice to offer other men trying to care for their wives, he had two suggestions: "Remember your two V's, Vows and Values. Honor them and have an agenda to follow every day. I always have something to follow."

Mr. Hansen and Mr. Gimmel represent the type of husband who oriented his caregiving role around the world of work. Caregiving became their new work identity for them, and they adapted to it with a renewed sense of purpose. They set up their "caregiving offices" and scheduled their days around caregiving duties. They relied on their old work skills to help them adapt to their new tasks.

"The Labor of Love"

This group of men are performing their caregiving duties as a labor of love. They acclimated to the caregiver role by merging it with their deep feelings toward their wives. Most of the men talked a great deal about their love for their wives and could express emotions easily. Much of the conversation was emotionally laden. For other men in this group, it was their actions that demonstrated this love: As they started to talk about their wives, the eyes would become moist and the throat tighten up. Some of these husbands spent a large portion of their time holding their wives' hands or with their arms around their wives. Many of them provided the hands-on care their wives needed. They looked at their wives and saw them as they were when they married. The caring for their wives was done out of devotion, not duty.

Mr. Stinholz

Mr. Stinholz is a small, trim, 68-year-old white man who retired from his accounting job five years ago. He has been caring for his wife for the past 10 years in their modest three-bedroom home. His house was neat and orderly. His wife is in the last stage of the disease. She is no longer able to walk, and has been unable to talk for three years.

When we first saw Mr. Stinholz, he had just finished feeding his wife breakfast, which is a lengthy process. He admitted, "It takes a long time, but I read the paper and I do my crossword puzzle. I don't just sit, it isn't a total drag for three hours; I enjoy myself being with my wife." Mr. Stinholz purchased a hospital bed, which he has placed in their living room so he can keep her close to him during the day.

Mr. Stinholz expresses the great loss he feels for his wife:

I miss most not being able to share the past with her or talk about a lot of things; we can't do it. I feel badly; we worked our life together to retire and travel and have a lot of fun together, and it's not working out. When I am home, I spend almost all my time sitting with her. We sit on the couch next to each other.

His wife still responds to affection; often, if she becomes agitated, to calm her down, he will sit beside her with his arm around her or hold her hand for hours. Mr. Stinholz also expresses his need for her tenderness and affection, "What I miss most is female companionship. I really miss our conversations. Women are just more compassionate and I just really miss that."

Near the end of the interview, Mr. Stinholz took us upstairs to show some earlier pictures of his wife. It was very important to him that we have a sense of who his wife was, not is. He had turned his den into a picture gallery of the life he has had with her, starting with a huge wedding picture, the first picture you notice as you enter the room. They have been married for 42 years; this picture gallery spans these years, marking the high points of their life together, from their engagement to the present. As Mr. Stinholz says, "I love her very much."

Mr. Stinholz built regular respite care into his life. He says, "I have set up a pretty good system of caring for my wife. I wouldn't enjoy it if I spent a hundred percent of my time with her." A paid caregiver comes into the home 20 hours a week, and every few months he leaves for a week to visit one of their six children, who live all over the United States. He shared his experience, saying, "You've got to take care of yourself, go out and do things you enjoy. If I fall apart, her system goes all to hell. Now my kids are good kids, but my wife is my problem. She's not the kids' problem."

Mr. Stinholz joined a newly formed all-male support group soon after his wife's diagnosis. He found the group extremely helpful, and recommends this to others.

I felt so devastated when I first found out about it. I thought my life was over. I started to feel sorry for myself. I didn't feel free to vent my feelings in other support groups that were probably fifty percent women. At our group there was a lot of integrity and on occasion guys would cry and nobody thought they were less of a man for doing it. I felt much freer. It turned my life around. I decided that I have a situation that I can do nothing about. I can make it more comfortable for my wife and myself, but I can't stop this thing, or change it or improve it. I've got to make the best of it.

Mr. Quiddly
As I pulled up into the driveway of Mr. Quiddly's small bungalow in a working-class section of town for the interview, I could not help

but notice his huge Harley-Davidson motorcycle resting against the side of the house. Mr. Quiddly opened the door, with his motorcycle jacket on; he had just returned from visiting his wife in the nursing home, where he had placed her three weeks earlier. His home was untidy and in need of attention.

Mr. Quiddly is a tall, slender, wiry white man of 73 years, caring for his wife in the middle stage of Alzheimer's disease. Prior to his wife's illness, he taught classes on auto mechanics. He was feeling quite guilty about his decision to place his wife in a nursing home. He admitted with much anguish that it was the hardest thing he ever had to do.

In caring for her, he injured his back, and this "scared him." Mr. Quiddly said, "I can't run the risk anymore of getting hurt again," but he deeply missed his wife and expressed his loss for her.

I'm so close to her, that body that's always been ours, mine, we share. I wish my little girl was back with me. I know the heartache and grief that is involved. I'm not eating very good now. I'm never very hungry now; I eat because I have to. I don't like eating my meals alone.

He was going every day to visit her in the nursing home. That morning he had just come back from having lunch with her. His discussion with me always came back to the topic of wondering whether she missed him.

Mr. Quiddly is trying to keep himself busy, reconnecting with activities he enjoyed before his wife became ill. Before the nursing home placement, he spent all his time taking care of his wife. He has started to ride his motorcycle again, is going roller-skating, and even went to the car races, but his thoughts always came back to his wife:

I'm back to what I did before, but I'm doing it all by myself. I do it to get my thoughts off my wife. And when I come home at night, I fall into bed . . . alone. I don't like it at all. I love my little girl. I do it because I have no choice.

Mr. Quiddly found support groups very helpful in sorting through his feelings. He recommends some type of support group to other husband caregivers:

I would encourage anybody to attend a meeting. I think everybody varies how much they get out of it. There are those that come and break down and weep. They either don't come back because they're embarrassed, because they thought they might have kind of, you know, displayed some emotion they shouldn't have. That isn't the case, or they'll come back because they find, here's a group who understands.

But it's his faith in God that has provided him the most solace during this caregiving experience:

Of all the things that saved the day, it's the faith in God I have. I understand God is sovereign. I'll never matter a matter to him. That doesn't matter if I don't understand. Even if I go to church and ask the question, "Why me?" That's not the question we should ask God. We should say, "What do you want me to learn from my experience to make me a better person?"

In response to my question, "Did it make you a better person," he replied, "I think so. I think I now have the ability to weep with those that weep, rejoice with those that rejoice, and to share with others."

Mr. Hastings

Mr. Hastings—a tall, quiet, and dignified white 76-year-old— was waiting for me at the door as I pulled into his driveway. Eleven years earlier he had retired from his job as director of a not-for-profit foundation to care for his wife. She was now 68 years old, and was diagnosed 12 years ago with early onset Alzheimer's disease. For Mr. Hastings, his actions often more than his words bespoke his commitment and love for his wife. He had designed the home for the sole purpose of caring for his wife; they had been living there for just one year. He was very proud of this accomplishment, and early in the interview he asked if I would like a tour of their home. The day I was there, his wife was in the hospital recuperating from a skin infection that required treatment with intravenous antibiotics. Mr. Hastings took me through every nook and cranny of the house, discussing how he had thought out the design of each feature of every room so his wife could be comfortable and he could give her the best care possible. Though now in the later stage of Alzheimer's disease, Mrs. Hastings was still able to walk, and her husband was determined to have her keep her mobility as long as possible. The design of the house aided in this endeavor.

During the interview, he brought me a picture of his wife taken when he first met her, when she was 20 years old. She was in nursing school and was wearing her new uniform. He recounted their meeting:

We met back when I was in college. I was starting my third year and she was the college nurse. She went to a hospital diploma nursing school; there were not many bachelor's nurses at the time, because there were not many places to get a bachelor's degree. So the college was taking nurses from her school and said, "If you want to be the school nurse, we'll give you room and board and your tuition, and you can get a bachelor's degree." I went back to school after the war and came down with malaria I contracted while in the army. I had seen it thousands of times. I knew exactly what it was. So I went down to the infirmary and here is this very pretty young nurse and I said, "I have malaria and I need quinine. Will you get me some quinine?" and I'll never forget, she said, "What makes you think you have malaria?" The old doctor there took one look at me and told her to give me the quinine. She said, "What's it like?" She had never seen any one with malaria. I said, "I'll tell you. It occurs every forty-eight hours. Just be prepared in two days and I'll give you a phone call. If you want to see it, come to my room. Bring your thermometer, and just watch," and she did. She always laughed about it saying, "I never saw such a thing in all my life," because my temperature went up to over a hundred and six, and I had chills that were so violent that it shook the bunk bed I was in. She sat there utterly amazed at what she was seeing.

Mr. Hastings was now providing total care to his wife. The only thing she could do unassisted was to feed herself a little breakfast. He talked about his new role:

If I gave her orange juice in a small glass, she could drink that. And drink a cup of coffee occasionally. Otherwise she does nothing. I dress her, bathe her, walk her around. I take her grocery shopping. I put her hands on the cart and put mine over them and we slowly walk around. I do all the cooking. I do all the laundry. I did all the cleaning until about four months ago. I had an aortic aneurism repaired. That sort of

took the pep out of me. So, I hired some cleaning ladies to come in. I
won't put her in a nursing home. She would have kept me home. She'd
live up to her responsibility if the role had been reversed.

Unlike other individuals with the disease, though, Mrs. Hastings
knew that she had Alzheimer's disease; in fact, she was the first one
to diagnose her condition. In all her nursing books and medical
books, she underlined the information on the disease. She also col-
lected newspaper clippings on the subject. So, after a series of diag-
nostic tests, when the doctor wanted to take Mr. Hastings aside to
tell him the results, Mrs. Hastings had already guessed. Mr. Hastings
said, "My wife told the doctor, I can tell you what is wrong with
me.' And when he said, 'What?' she said, 'I am an Alzheimer's patient. I read all the books and decided that's what was wrong with
me.' Now this was back in the early eighties when not many people
knew about Alzheimer's. And the doctor said, 'I think you are right.'
She was a lady with a high I.Q., so I wasn't surprised."

Mr. Hastings was very lonely. He missed immensely the relationship he had with his wife previous to the disease. They had a
very deep, caring relationship, based upon mutual respect and love,
and he felt a great sense of loss. As he talked about their relationship,
his eyes became moist and his voice softened:

The most difficult thing for me is to watch my wife deteriorate, because
we did everything together. I never went on a vacation by myself. Sel-
dom did either of us go anyplace without the other. I don't know if that's
good or bad, but we didn't. If she wanted to go shopping for clothes, I
went with her. And I enjoyed it. If I wanted to go fishing, she'd go with
me. I always enjoyed having her with me. Always, always, always.

After pausing to collect his emotions, Mr. Hastings continued:

We have always been positively the best of friends. I used to be able to
come home from work, and I could have had the world's worst day. I
would come in the house, and my wife would be cooking, and I'd sit
down in the kitchen and I would sound off, going through my day. It
might take half an hour, but just really bare my soul. And I think back
at it; what she did was listen. She didn't advise me. She never said she

*would help me or anything like that, or do this or do that. She truly
listened. And that was really all that was necessary.*

Adding to Mr. Hastings' loneliness was his feeling of being socially isolated. He had a sister living near by who was very helpful
and often provided some brief needed respite for him. His two children lived out of town and were as helpful and concerned as they
could be; but most of their friends had disappeared. Most of their
friends they had met through his wife, and when that tie was loos-
ened, they drifted apart. Mr. Hastings commented, "It's very difficult and it sort of hurts. I've found strangers to be very helpful once
you explain the situation . . . everybody except your real friends. There
are even people on this street. We've only been here a year and they
would stop me and ask me how my wife is doing."

Attending a support group has particularly helped Mr. Hastings
cope with his situation and his wife's deteriorating condition. He
reflected back on his initial reaction to a support group and how it
has helped him.

*When I first went [to a group], I didn't find it helpful. I thought, "Why
should I sit here and listen to other people's problems? I've got my own
without listening to theirs." And now it has truly helped. I had a difficult decision to make one day. I found my wife on her hands and knees
in the dressing room. And I was trying to determine what to do. And I
chose to leave her, and she went to sleep standing up, and fell down
gracefully. I should have gotten her up, but I was afraid I would hurt
her and me, but afterwards I felt very guilty. So I talked to the people
there; I opened the meeting. And now it's probably the biggest help. I
have other difficult choices to make. I truly think the Alzheimer's groups
are very helpful if you can get past the point of "I don't want to listen to
everyone else's troubles.". . . I just listen to somebody else and realize that
you're not the only one with lots of problems. I think sharing common
experiences with someone makes it easier.*

Mr. Hastings, like Mr. Stinholz and Mr. Quiddly, well represented
the type of husband caregiver who oriented his caregiving role around
the theme of love for his wife. Thus, these husbands were labeled
"labor of love." Through their words and actions, all three men ex-

pressed this deep devotion to their wives. The sense of loss for their closest friend, companion, and their lover was profound. The sense of social isolation felt was extreme. Often they found some comfort in attending a support group where they could share their feelings and establish some bonds of common fellowship.

"Sense of Duty"

"Sense of duty" husbands felt an intensely developed sense of responsibility in caring for their wives. They oriented to the caregiving role by focusing on this sense of duty. Their discussions on caregiving focused on commitment, duty, and responsibility. They would not desert their responsibility of caring for their wives.

Mr. Jones

Mr. Jones is a tall, stately looking 73-year-old African-American man who is a strong presence when he enters a room. He had begun training as a minister, but decided he could not make that commitment. As he said, "You can't cheat on the Maker," so he worked as a truck driver for a food distributor for many years. His dignified demeanor was in sharp contrast to his appearance: an unshaven face and shirt tails hanging out of his pants.

Last year he and his wife moved into their daughter's home in the suburbs so their daughter could help with the care of her mother. Leaving his own home and neighborhood was a very difficult move for Mr. Jones.

My daughter began pestering me to get out of Cleveland. "Come on, Dad. I'll help you." And I guess she does, but she travels a lot with her job. She is the executive director of a large association. Only thing about it is we ain't too compatible. She feels, she has a Ph.D. and I have nothin'.

Mrs. Jones is in the middle stage of Alzheimer's disease. She smiles appropriately, though she can no longer hold a conversation. She can say only a few words. Mr. Jones mentioned that she used to wander—he had lost her two times—though she does not wander anymore. Throughout the course of the interview, Mrs. Jones sat quietly at the kitchen table folding and unfolding her napkin.

Mr. Jones is strongly committed to caring for his wife of 43 years:

As long as these two weak knees can move one step in front of another, I will care for her. I made a vow to this woman and I intend to keep it. Don't matter if she would do it for me. I know what I need to do, and so does the man upstairs.

For Mr. Jones, the most difficult part of taking care of his wife is helping with her personal care needs. He finds getting her dressed particularly difficult, though he has learned the "tricks of the trade":

Forget about stockings. Forget about skirt. Forget about blouses. Just give her some decent slacks to put on and it comes in handy if you take her to the john. If she got all that fancy stuff on, I guarantee you the next day you will do it differently.

He has also had to take over balancing the checkbook, which he had never done in his life. As he said, "That was her job. I'd come home and put the money on the table and say, 'Here.' Now I have to pay the bills."

One day a week Mrs. Jones attends a nearby adult day care program. When asked if she seems to enjoy the activity, Mr. Jones is unsure: "I just don't know if she enjoys it. You just don't know."

I was very much struck by Mr. Jones's philosophical and spiritual approach to his caregiving experience; he saw it as part of life and realized that one gets used to it. Talking about his faith, he said, "Every day it helps me to understand a lot of stuff that I didn't understand. It gives me an insight." He has accepted his lot in life, but at times feels as though he has been cheated.

We used to travel a lot, you know. We've been to Hawaii twice, been to the Bahamas half a dozen times and we were getting ready to go to Europe when this thing happened. Some things we meant to do together, we didn't get a chance to do.

Mr. Jones still manages to get out with his wife. He enjoys fishing, and in the spring and summer takes his wife with him often. He takes a lawn chair and sits his wife right next to him as he fishes. She will sit there for hours with him, not saying a word.

Offering advice to other husbands who are beginning to care for their wives with dementia, Mr. Jones had some words of wisdom:

Tell them the truth, that you are going to have to do it. It's a very diffi-cult road and they're gonna have to make some changes. Slow down the pace. You have to watch most things to make sure you're not wearing the person down. Then you have to make those times count.

Mr. O'Neal

Mr. O'Neal had traveled and moved many times in his life. His work as a seismologist had literally taken him to the four corners of the earth. Sometimes his wife and children moved with him, and other times they stayed behind. Now, with his wife's recent diagno-sis of Alzheimer's disease at age 68, they moved into a retirement community. The decorations in their house reflect his international voyages, particularly his years in South America, but this move was the most difficult for this 70-year-old white adventurer.

Mr. O'Neal accepts responsibility for his wife, but it is mingled with much resentment:

There is only one reason we moved here [to the life care community]. I don't want to, to put it bluntly, change her diapers later on. So that is why we wanted a place. Is that blunt enough? . . . So here we are for life. They will help me take care of her, which is a relief. You don't have to worry about it.

Mr. O'Neal selected this particular facility for them to live in because of the full range of services it offers, especially when his wife needs more assistance. At the moment, they are living in a beautiful house with cathedral ceilings that he designed himself. It is clearly one of the largest and most beautiful homes in the community, of which he is very proud, but he talked also about the time when her dementia would require they move into an apartment. Out of his sense of duty to his wife, he is committed to remain with her and make sure her care is provided. He knew he could plan for and con-trol only so much: "I'm sure there will be things that come up, but I haven't spent time dwelling on them. I thought more or less, I've gone as far as I could when I moved here. Whatever goes on from here goes on."

For Mr. O'Neal, freedom and independence were very important, and this facility allowed him to maintain this. He could drop his wife off at a community activity and have some time to himself. One of his major coping strategies is woodworking. He set up an elaborate woodworking shop in his basement, and could stay there eight hours a day working on one of his furniture designs, forgetting about his wife's situation. At this time, the most difficult aspect of the disease for the two of them to handle is Mrs. O'Neal's forgetfulness and repetitive questioning. As Mr. O'Neal said, "She can't remember what you would tell her in two seconds." Mrs. O'Neal, who had joined us in their living room, responded, "I would go around asking the same questions over and over again." Mr. O'Neal continued, "Yeah. I'd have to answer what day it is over and over again. Boy, did they make a big mistake. They gave her the happy pill and they ought to give it to the husband."

Attending a specialized short-term support group for early diagnosed individuals and their family members was very helpful for the O'Neals. Mr. O'Neal expressed his gratitude toward this group:

The one thing I appreciate about them [the support group] is it finally convinced her that it is better to admit it [having Alzheimer's disease]. Tell people you got it; it's better than running around trying to hide it. And she's been a whole lot happier since it's occurred.

Discussing her reaction to their recent move and her illness, Mrs. O'Neal shared with us, "Well, it is not easy. He's done the best he can for me. So I go along with it. I can't fight for myself anymore." There is a family history of the illness. Mrs. O'Neal's brother was diagnosed with Alzheimer's, and he died 10 years ago.

Near the end of the interview, Mr. O'Neal summed up his thoughts about his wife's disease, "This isn't anybody's fault. It just happened. Period. Accept it."

Mr. Bishop

Mr. Bishop is a soft-spoken, distinguished 71-year-old African-American whose manner could be described as one of quiet forbearance. He is a man of few words. He is a well-educated man, and had worked at one of the government space agencies before retiring. He was dressed very comfortably in a red-checkered flannel shirt and a pair of jeans held up by suspenders. He apologized for his appearance, and said he needs to dress comfortably to care for his wife. He is held in high esteem by his daughter, son-in-law, and their two children, who live with him. This three-generation family lives in a cozy home in an integrated suburban community.

Mr. Bishop and his wife have been married for 50 years; 10 years ago she was diagnosed with Alzheimer's. In 1989, she experienced a major stroke that, together with her end-stage Alzheimer's, left her bedridden, unable to communicate, and in need of a feeding tube. Mr. Bishop provides all the hands-on care to his wife, accepting little assistance from others. He sees it as his responsibility. There is a respite worker, a home health aide, who comes twice a month for a few hours to relieve him, but he is very particular about whom he allows to help his wife. His daughter does the cooking and housecleaning, and his son-in-law maintains the upkeep of the house. On the day of our interview, the son-in-law had taken a day off from work to help Mr. Bishop lay a new kitchen floor.

For Mr. Bishop, the most difficult part of his caregiving responsibilities is the lifting. He described his difficulties:

Lifting is the worst part. Before the stroke, she was a well-trimmed person. She was very particular about her weight, but since her stroke she put on weight. It takes a lot of energy to move her, bathe her, change her, get her into position to feed her. I feed her four times a day and up and down the steps. It is a regular routine for me now. The only thing is that I get tired a little bit. But one of my daughters lives with me, has ever since she got married, so I get a little chance to relax. She has a new baby, though.

Another difficulty that frustrates Mr. Bishop is his own arthritis, which interferes with providing the kind of care he would like to give his wife:

I started some exercises with her [his wife] some time ago, and then I gave up on that; but I've gone back to exercising her again. But the exercising increases my soreness in my arms and so forth. Plus I have arthritis in my knees, and that bugs me.

Mr. Bishop has been very resourceful, installing mechanical aids to help him provide care for his wife. He installed a wheelchair ramp, a bathtub lift, and a chair lift for the stairs. He takes much pride in these accomplishments. He decided those were the things he needed to provide quality care. The tub lift has been a big assistance for him in bathing her, and the chair lift allows him to take his wife downstairs, so she can still be part of the family. He keeps a hospital bed in the living room for her, among the television and video games that his grandson uses. His three daughters and son helped him to purchase the chair lift. He talked about their help:

I knew the stair glide would be easier on me if I would purchase that. The fact of the matter is, my daughter, the second oldest, had the idea that all of my daughters and my son pitch in together to make the original investment. So, that wasn't all an expense on me. So we paid it off.

Each day, Mr. Bishop asks his wife if she wants to go downstairs in the afternoon after her nap. He understands her by her facial expressions. During our interview, when I went upstairs to meet Mrs. Bishop, her face lit up when her husband entered the room. He said, "Yes, she knows me, yes. If someone is here with us she looks to me to explain what is going on."

His grandchildren have accepted their grandmother's condition as part of life. They have always lived with their grandparents and really have no other memory of their grandmother. When the grandchildren come back from school in the afternoon, they go over to their grandmother and give her a kiss. Mr. Bishop stated matter-of-factly, "My grandchildren have accepted it, as have my children; even my son, who had the most difficult time. They know the situation and respond to it."

What primarily has helped Mr. Bishop cope with his caregiving responsibilities is his deep sense of commitment and responsibility toward his wife, as well as his overall philosophy of life. He shared his thoughts, saying, "Why do I do it? It goes back to my basic philosophy. This is part of life, and she would have done the same thing for me. My mother did it for her mother, and I will never abandon her." He continued after a long pause and reflected, "My life has been fair. I learned a great deal from her [his wife]. She was a nurse, and I learned to take care of people from her. I'll take one day at a time. Whatever happens tomorrow, I'll do the best that I can."

He does find some time away once in a while to go fishing, which he finds very enjoyable and relaxing. We discussed the salmon fishing expedition he took a few weeks ago with his son-in-law, when he caught one of the largest salmons he ever caught. When he goes away, his children pitch in to help care for their mother, though as Mr. Bishop said, "I don't like to ask them too much."

He misses the trips that they had planned to take together after he retired. He sadly said:

We were going to drive from this side of the country to the other, from the south all the way to the north. I had plans of taking my wife to England once, going over seas to Israel and Europe. I went with my work and wanted to take her, but she didn't want to go while the kids were in school, so she stayed home.

He misses the former life he had with his wife, yet like many of the husbands who have been caregiving for their wives a long time, he finds some positive aspects in the experience. He shared, "I think I am a little more patient now, a little bit more tolerant of . . . others. In fact, I try not to be a burden to others, especially my family."

I asked him if he had any advice he would share with other husbands caring for wives with dementia at home; he pondered for a while and then quietly said:

I think they have to look at Alzheimer's in a certain frame of mind to be able to go with the flow. You can't think negatively about Alzheimer's. For example, I don't think about my wife's death at all. I'm glad I am able to do for her. I feel she would do the same for me. I'm sure there are times when you are feeling down, but a prayer and a little fishing always helps. You have to take a day at a time and do the best that you can do to take care of her.

Mr. Bishop, Mr. O'Neal, and Mr. Jones typify the type of husband caregiver we named "sense of duty." They feel a deep sense of responsibility to care for their wives. They expressed this sentiment often during the course of the interview. Sometimes they provided the hands-on care to their wives, and sometimes they hired someone to provide that care, but they saw taking care of their wives as their duty.

"Going It Together"

Caregiving for this group of men was a team approach. Their wives were in the early stage of dementia and could still plan and participate in their own care. Decisions about the future were joint ones, as they had always been during their years of marriage. Not all wives in the early stage of dementia are cognitively aware enough or strong enough to face the challenges that lie ahead of them; however, these couples were able to do just that together. It is uncertain how long they would be able to use this type of orientation in handling the wife's illness, but until her dementia impaired her judgment and cognitive ability, these couples would work jointly. This did not mean that the wife did not have mild periods of confusion and forgetfulness, but these couples were able to work around these times.

Mr. and Mrs. Jenko

Mr. and Mrs. Jenko are learning to handle this disease together. Mrs. Jenko has early onset dementia, diagnosed 18 months ago at the age of 43. She is no longer able to handle her bookkeeping job, and even her love for tap dancing has been interrupted, as she has difficulty remembering the routines; she has a positive outlook, however, and a wonderful sense of humor.

Mr. Jenko is a white 41-year-old truck driver of slight build, a quiet reflective man who tries to approach life in a logical, orderly fashion. Previously he saw the world only in terms of black and white; there was no room for shades of gray. His wife's illness has caused him to reevaluate his view on life. It is a second marriage for both of them, and Mr. Jenko is devoted to caring for his wife. Mrs. Jenko has three children in their late teens and early twenties who have moved back into the house. They have rearranged their schedules so that Mrs. Jenko is not left alone.

As I entered their small, cozy home, both Mr. and Mrs. Jenko were waiting for me in their living room. Mrs. Jenko was uncertain whether she would be welcome to participate in the interview, but both were visibly relieved when assured that her participation was to

be their decision. Upon receiving this information, they both relaxed and started to tell me their story.

They told their story together, and Mr. Jenko often assisted his
wife by finishing her sentences, as she had difficulty finding the right
words to express her thoughts and feelings. She found this assistance
a great relief. She in turn helped him to express feelings about their
situation that he had trouble discussing.

Because of Mrs. Jenko's young age, the diagnosis of dementia
was a long, drawn-out, difficult period in their lives. Mr. Jenko discussed some of the frustrations he experienced while waiting for his
wife's symptoms to be diagnosed and given a name.

*Our lives were definitely coming apart. No matter which way we counted,
it seemed like there was no way to pull it back together again. I felt bad for
her because I knew what she used to be like and even with some of the
simple daily things, you know, like a pot of tea or something like that. She
would get stuck, and I was as guilty as the rest of them. I would say, "Come
on, just do it; how the hell hard can it be to make a cup of tea."*

He has had to readjust his entire worldview to work together
with his wife.

*I've definitely learned to look at this a whole lot differently. Things that
she used to do every day, I took for granted. I can't do it anymore. She
used to yell at me all the time because I am black or white. There is no
gray, you know. It's either right or wrong, or it's up or down. Now I can't
get away from that damn color gray. I hate gray.*

Mr. Jenko has also had to reprioritize his life. His work always
came first, and then his family. The whole family now works together to maintain strong ties and "be there for each other."

*I'll tell you, I am not the sweetest guy in the world. I've got to be one of
the hardest people to live with because, up until recently, my job came
first, then my family, because without a job, I wouldn't have a family.
So, now it's the opposite. It's my family, then my job. My biggest priority
is to make her happy, because only God knows how much more time I'm
going to have with her, and I want it to be happy.*

Together they have worked out a system to help care for Mrs. Jenko. Mrs. Jenko reads all sorts of information on behavior management of someone with dementia. She then shares this information with her husband, which better equips him to handle her when she exhibits symptoms such as agitation and forgetfulness. It is definitely a team approach, as illustrated by the conversation below:

Mrs. Jenko: *I read somewhere that when your memory starts to go or something, your habits will take over.*

Mr. Jenko: *Right. So with my job, I start at all hours. I used to just set the alarm, get up and go to work and then I would come home when I finished. Now, what I do is leave her a note and I put down where I'm going, what time I left the house and the date. I always leave the date because she has a hard time with memory.*

They gave another example of this approach.

Mr. Jenko: *If we're in the house and she starts to get agitated or argumentative, I kind of sneak in the back door and change the subject, and I try to distract her. This usually seems to help because she will calm down. A lot of these things I learn from her because she would tell me, "Look I've read all the stuff from the Alzheimer's Association. They say to do this stuff." And I don't have time to read that stuff.*

Mrs. Jenko: *I did! I said, "Here's what you need to do because I'm not going to be able to remind you when I need it," and it's true. It worked out, I have every book there is on Alzheimer's.*

One of the most disturbing aspects of the disease that both Mr. and Mrs. Jenko have had to deal with is the limited support they have received from friends and extended family members. Her extended family could not accept the diagnosis. Mrs. Jenko commented, "It's been a real rough road." As for friends, she said, "My friends? My friends are now. . . ." "Gone," said Mr. Jenko, completing the sentence. "Yes, but," said Mrs. Jenko, "they have been replaced with fellow travelers."

These "fellow travelers" are members of a specialized support group for early diagnosed individuals and their family members (attended by Mr. and Mrs. Jenko). They found this experience very beneficial for both of them, and when the group officially ended, they still continued to meet. As Mrs. Jenko stated, "They are the best friends I have ever had."

This experience with dementia has brought this couple closer together, and in their own words, "has been a mixed blessing." Mrs. Jenko commented, "You know, maybe it has [brought them closer]. Maybe that is why I'm much more happy, because it seems like nothing in my life is working anymore, but everything is working right. So in all essence, as dumb as it sounds, . . ." "It has brought us closer," concluded Mr. Jenko.

When asked to suggest some words of advice for other husbands caring for a wife with dementia, he offered these thoughts:

I think the most important piece of advice I could give them is look at how they used to be, not the way they are now and ask yourself why it's not like that and what you can do. That and be kind. Expect very little and be overexuberant with what you get and they won't go far wrong. And most of all, learn to listen.

Turning to his wife, he said, "What do you think?" And Mrs. Jenko stated, "I think that sounds nice."

Mr. and Mrs. Plastoff

Mr. and Mrs. Plastoff are also able to talk about their situation together. Mrs. Plastoff is 77 years old, 4 years older than her husband, and is in the early stage of dementia. Both of them admit that she has her good days and her bad days. They have been married for 52 years and live in a comfortable home in a predominantly white working-class community, and their children live nearby. Mr. Plastoff owned a gas station downtown for many years, but sold it when the neighborhood began to deteriorate.

The diagnosis of Alzheimer's disease has been devastating for him, and his wife is helping him to deal with it as well as herself. He was visibly agitated and wringing his hands. Mrs. Plastoff was more able to accept the changes she saw in herself. She said, "It's hard to swallow when you get it, but you get used to it." She actively participated in the interview, and was relieved to know that she would not be left out.

Mr. Plastoff spoke of first noticing the signs of dementia in his wife:

About four years ago, I began to notice things that weren't quite normal. The first thing I noticed was her penmanship. She had the most beautiful penmanship of anybody, and then it just got to the point where it was more like scribble. She, at times, even hesitates in writing her name.

Mrs. Plastoff continued, "It came to a point where I couldn't write my name. How could I not remember my last name?"

Mr. Plastoff confessed that the diagnosis "changed my world all around." He had never balanced a checkbook before or paid the bills. Now he is "stuck doing everything," even cooking, but at least they were able to talk about it. Mrs. Plastoff is able to voice much empathy for her husband. She can express feelings for him that he has difficulty verbalizing:

He knows what's happening with me and how far long gone I've gone, and how much I've deteriorated. That's what really hurts is the deterioration [speaking for both of them]. I can't remember people; even the day before I can't remember. And I know at first he used to get real antagonistic. He'd tell me and I would turn around and I'd ask him the same questions all over again. That makes you buggy pretty soon. And sometimes I'm real sharp with him too, and I don't like it.

Mr. Plastoff chimed in, "She picks on me." Mrs. Plastoff responded, "If I were only picking on him!"

For Mr. Plastoff, one of the most difficult parts of caring for his wife is his feeling of being tied down. He has lost his freedom, and this theme echoes throughout the interview.

The hardest thing to take for me is that they took her driving privileges away. Now, I have to take her wherever she wants to go, whenever. And I have to watch every move she makes. Before I went on my own pretty much.

Mrs. Plastoff adds, *"Definitely tied down, because he's never sure that I won't take off and take a walk."*

Friends and family have been very helpful and have given Mr. Plastoff some relief. They still go out with friends, though not as much as before. When they do, the wives "watch over" Mrs. Plastoff, so he has time with the men. They have informed their friends, neighbors, and family of the diagnosis to eliminate hiding or covering up instances of Mrs. Plastoff's unusual behavior. As for their children, Mr. Plastoff said, "They're all helpful. If I ask any one of them for help, they are right here."

The Plastoffs were also part of a support group for early diagnosed individuals and their families. This provided them with much support and prepared them to face the situation together. Mr. Plastoff expressed his thoughts about the group experience:

The support group helped us most of all because we got to meet a lot of people with the same problems that we had. Through the discussions and talks, we're all in the same boat. Things are happening to all of us in the same way.

Mrs. Plastoff also discussed her experience in the group:

Yes. It helped me to know—they talked to me. People stay out of your way, even though I'm a real good friend. You just have a feeling that they are afraid, afraid of getting it, or if they'll hurt my feelings. But you see when you went with them [came to the support group], they were all in the same boat and I could talk to them. There was the feeling that these people understood. You're not alone.

Mr. Plastoff's closing suggestion for other husbands caring for a wife with dementia was to join a support group for the early diagnosed where both of them could come together and discuss issues with people in similar circumstances. Mrs. Plastoff added, "Just tell them there are other people—they're laughing. They're still having fun. You don't lie down and die."

Mr. and Mrs. Rollins

Mr. Rollins is a small stocky, 83-year-old African-American man who retired 18 years ago from his maintenance job. He is in poor health and due to a severe back problem walks very slowly and painfully with the use of a crutch. He is recuperating presently from a recent heart attack. His wife, 76 years old, was diagnosed with early stage dementia six months ago. She too has severe cardiac and pulmonary health care problems that complicate managing her care. Mr. and Mrs. Rollins live in a four-room bungalow with broken front steps and a sagging porch badly in need of repair. Old newspapers are stacked all over their living room; housekeeping seems to have become an overwhelmimg chore. The recent diagnosis of dementia is yet one more stress this couple must deal with in their daily lives. Mr. Rollins commented, "To tell ya the truth, when people look at us, they say we are lucky to be here; but the Lord has blessed us and we are doin' the best that we can for each other."

Mr. Rollins is a proud, independent individual who worked all his life. He shared some of his early experiences:

I started to work when I was six years old. I worked the farm; I worked the saw mill; I worked the road. Me and my daddy worked. And if we weren't able to pay, we worked it out. He worked his and I worked mine, wherever I could get a job.

Mr. Rollins takes on life's challenges and meets them squarely in the face. He expressed his underlying philosophy early on in the course of the interview: "Where there is a will, there is a way; and I've tried to keep that will. When I can only go so far, she [his wife] will take it [over] and do the best that she can."

It was very important to Mr. Rollins that his wife be included and participate in our discussion. As soon as I entered the house, he asked if his wife could join us around the kitchen table and participate. It is very important to him that they work together. He stated clearly and strongly:

I feel we [he and his wife] can work together and understand each other. I can understand her and she can understand me. I didn't want you to

come and sit down and talk and not let her know what we were talkin'
about. You know what I mean? It might get to one day when someone
has to take care of me. We all gettin' to that age.

Mrs. Rollins knows she is getting forgetful, especially in the
kitchen, where she often leaves the stove burning. She does not have
a clear understanding of what is happening to her, though she knows
her memory is poor. Yet she is still trying to maintain some independence. She admitted, "You know I can't tell what the month is, but
I can still do for myself." Together they told their story. Mr. Rollins
started:

We are gettin' to that age now so where we don't know where we gonna
be tomorrow. We are here today. So, we just have to take it a day at a
time, a step at a time, and live the day. But I just pray and hope we be
able to stay together. It took me about three months or more to get her to
even say, "Yes" [to marry him]. When I told the judge "I will," that
meant as long as I live.

Mrs. Rollins interrupted him, saying, "She [the interviewer] doesn't
want to hear all that." And Mr. Rollins protested, "Hush woman, she
has come to hear what we both have to say." Mr. Rollins continued:

We ain't never been one to fight with one another. We might disagree,
but that's far as it goes. If she gets a little ornery, I ain't gonna say
nothin', and if I get that way, she ain't gonna say nothin', so it's all
done with!

Mrs. Rollins chimed in: "Oh, yeah, we have a good relationship.
Beautiful. You don't see it much these days." They helped each other
during difficult times. Both of them are struggling with trying to
understand Alzheimer's disease and the impact it will have on their
lives. Mr. Rollins commented:

There's been a lot of talk around people forgetting and drifting off. They
talkin' this and that, but the doctor he ain't never just sit down and
talked about it. And that's the big thing see, so I had to come out and ask
the questions because I want to know. See, she got a sister in Birming-

ham and she's in bad shape. So we want to know what's goin' on. I have a book here and I've been readin' it, but see I can't read all that good, but I can read enough to understand some. We know it's gonna get worse. So we together just have to be watchful and be careful, and so I try to read and understand it, and we discuss things. And if we don't fully get it, we just leave it alone.

Mrs. Rollins has started having some communication problems, such as finding the right word when she speaks, and this often frustrates her. Mr. Rollins tries to help her. He explains the situation and his role:

When she tries to bring out somethin', she can't bring it out. She'll get frustrated and others, they look like they're gettin' short of patience with her, and I tell 'em, "You all, I'm here with her all the time and I kinda picture the way she's talkin'." I try to bring in the words. I be lookin' to hit this nail on the head and she'll say, "That's what I'm trying to say."

I feel that we can work together and understand each other. I can understand her and she can understand me. You know what I mean?

The most difficult thing for the Rollinses to cope with now is the increasing cost of their medications and medical bills. Mr. Rollins has been turned down for Medicaid because of a small life insurance policy. They both are very upset about the situation. He is in the process of appealing the decision. Mr. Rollins angrily stated:

I done worked all my life and I can't work now. And now with all our bills that we have, we're just not able to get the proper medicine. And I told her [Mrs. Rollins], "Now, Honey, with that doctor appointment tomorrow, if it's any more expensive medicine, just say, NO!" We can't afford no more bills, and the Medicare just pays so much. That's the condition we in, so we have to be careful. We need medicine and stuff like that, but we just can't get it!

Mrs. Rollins nodded in agreement and added, "I wonder sometimes, why is that? I'm out of medicine right now and there ain't nothing I can do. I heard people tell lies about their money, but God knows I ain't gonna do that."

The two major supports for this elderly couple are their grandson, whom they raised, and their church. Their grandson works two jobs, but on Sundays, his day off, he comes to take his grandparents to church, 45 minutes from their house. Mrs. Rollins said about her grandson:

He's such a sweet child. He's a wonderful child. He always has been. The only somebody I can really depend upon is him. I got another grandson and granddaughter, but I don't know what to say about 'em sometime. They just ain't—you know, how young people are now. Some of 'em being on drugs, and you can't depend upon them no kinda way.

Mr. Rollins added:

Last week, I managed to slide the garbage out, but she's scared I might fall. I couldn't carry it. I just put it down and just slid it along in front of me on the curb. A young fella that I knew called me and I said, "Like on a Wednesday, you could call me, and I might give you a little somethin' to come and take the garbage out." When my grandson heard that, he said, "Listen, don't you do that. You call me, you know I might forget it, but leave it on my answering machine. When I get off from work, I'll come down and take care of it."

Religion is a central focus in their lives, and Mr. Rollins proudly told me he is a deacon of his church. Mr. Rollins confided, "I feel it's a blessin' to be a servant of the Lord. The Lord has blessed me because they chose me as their deacon." Mrs. Rollins discussed proudly her husband's hard work and dedication to their church. Not only does their religion provide them with spiritual support, it also is a source of strong social support. He is in close contact with a number of people from their congregation. Members of the congregation will check to see if the couple has enough food and heat. One young congregation member will come sometimes during the week and take them to a prayer meeting. Mrs. Rollins stated, "That young woman is like a daughter to us." During the course of the interview, three church members called to talk to Mr. Rollins, to check on the couple and ask for advice.

Mr. and Mrs. Rollins, Mr. and Mrs. Plastoff, and Mr. and Mrs. Jenko illustrate the "going it together" type of caregiver. Orienting to caregiving for this group of men was achieved through team effort. Their wives were able to participate in the planning of their care, and decisions were made jointly, as they always had been in the course of their marriages. The husbands helped their wives when they became forgetful, or agitated, or frustrated; the wives helped their husbands deal with the impact the disease was having on both of them. They were a source of strength and mutual support for each other.

"Men in Transition"

The "men in transition" caregivers are usually new to caregiving, or men whose wives have just moved into a new stage in the downward spiral of dementia. They are in transition from their previous roles as husband and provider to their new role as caregiver. This change takes place on two levels: a surface level, where husbands are learning new skills and trying to decide what the best course of action is; and a more psychological level, where the men deeply feel this transition and the changes that must take place in themselves and their wives. Some of these "men in transition" caregivers exhibit more of one level than the other.

Men dealing mainly with the first level are floundering among the choices of what to do next. Their conversations focus on exploring different options and roads to take in caring for their wives, including the dilemmas they themselves face. They also speak of their frustrations and exhibit caregiver stress, as is illustrated by the two narratives below.

Mr. Kerns

Mr. Kerns is a young-looking, physically fit 67-year-old business executive and lawyer who recently retired. His life had previously centered around his work. His wife, also 67 years old, is in the early stage of dementia, slowly moving into the middle stage. They have been married for over 40 years and live in a luxury home in a wealthy suburb. They have two daughters who both live out of town, but talk with them on a regular basis. He uses day care services for his wife twice a week, and a housekeeper several times a month.

At the time of the interview, Mr. Kerns was in a state of crisis. He was at a crossroads. His wife was becoming worse and he had not set up any routine system of care for her changing condition. He was feeling overwhelmed.

You don't know where the hell to start. God, it's just totally frustrating to have nowhere to turn, nowhere to go, just nothing, but I said, "If that's it, I've got to live with it."

Mr. Kerns used to be able to leave his wife alone at home for a couple of hours, but now was unable to do so. During much of the interview he discussed different options for providing care, mainly companionship, for his wife. He was thinking out his plan of action. Below are two examples:

Here is the dilemma; I have to start making arrangements, you know, someone to be her companion while I go here or there or somewhere else. I have to deal with it. It is so frustrating, she is so young. Up to last year, I could leave her alone for a couple of hours, and in a crunch I would utilize some very close friends, but I know this is not good.

He continued later in the interview, saying:

I really have a great difficulty. So, if it got to the point that required full-time around-the-clock care, I'm gonna have a damn tough decision. I'm not sure which way it's gonna go at this point in time. Having in-home care gives you more flexibility, but I'd probably say right now if I had to make a decision, "Hey, put her into a nursing home," for my own sanity and peace of mind.

They are still both physically active. Mrs. Kerns can still ride a bike, which they do often in the city parks near their home. They enjoy short car rides together, and on occasion take their van out of town to visit their daughters. As long as Mr. Kerns is close by, and she can see him, Mrs. Kerns is comfortable in unfamiliar surroundings. If he gets out of sight, "she panics."

Mr. Kerns has learned to cook, out of self-preservation, he says, and to handle other housekeeping chores. But for him, one of the "toughest" aspects of this caregiving role is the social isolation. He did not find the two support group meetings he attended to be beneficial. He felt, "I have my own headaches. I don't have to listen to other people's misery. I guess I have not got a great deal out of the support group in the sense of something that I can say, "Hey, this really helped me."

He particularly misses the socialization with his former business associates and colleagues. He stills tries to attend the monthly luncheon meetings of an investment group formed by former co-workers, but even this is getting more difficult to attend because of his wife's changing condition.

Mr. Kerns's suggestion for helping men deal with the situation of caring for an ill wife reflects this isolation.

I don't know if there's any way of really dealing with this situation of your friends and associates, but if there was some way of educating these people, or getting some sort of seminars or material into their hands . . . maybe a program devoted to friends of people with Alzheimer's. Those who attend would have a heck of a lot better understanding.

Mr. Martin

The long, winding dirt road leading down to the Martins' house was full of potholes and large puddles. The house is one of four situated on an isolated rural road. The small bungalow sits a quarter-mile from any neighbors, and 70 miles from a major urban area. It took Mr. Martin three hours round trip to drive to work and back from the auto plant before he retired nine years ago. He was very proud of the house that he built with his own hands 17 years ago, and until recently, never regretted moving out to the country to raise his family.

As I entered their home, Mr. Martin was cooking lunch for his wife, hot dogs and soup, and he politely offered me a platter. There were piles of bills and other papers stacked on the floor next to what seemed to be his favorite chair. Their dining room table was also filled with what looked like medical bills.

Mr. Martin is a small, tense 59-year-old African-American man of slight build with a fierce sense of pride and independence. His

wife was diagnosed nine years ago at the age of 51 with early onset
Alzheimer's disease. Now, for the first time in his life, he is in need of
help, yet does not want to ask for it. His wife is moving into the
middle stage of the disease and is becoming completely dependent
upon him. She is a very beautiful woman who was the valedictorian
of her high school class. Mr. Martin was very proud of his wife's past
accomplishments and confided, "You know there was nothing my
wife didn't know before she got sick. I'm a crossword puzzle buff. I
like to do crosswords. I never had to use a dictionary before she got
sick." Now during our interview, Mrs. Martin could only partially
follow the conversation.

Mr. Martin's whole life has been turned upside down. He explained, "Until 1905, I wasn't spending too much time at home. I
was working 12-hour days, and it was taking me an hour and a half
to get there and an hour and a half to come home. I just wasn't home
that much. Understand what I'm saying?" Now Mr. Martin has a
completely new role. He confided, "I do washing, ironing, cooking,
taking care of my wife. We've been married 38 years. I never boiled
a wiener before . . . no, I never even boiled a wiener before." In a
resigned, flat voice with little affect he continued, "And now, we are
just here all the time. Ninety-nine percent of the time when I run
out, I got my wife with me, 'cause I can't leave her by herself."

Another major issue that Mr. Martin was struggling with was
the ever-mounting medical and hospital bills for his wife. The dilemma of handling her health care expenditures was overwhelming
Mr. Martin. The bills, in various piles in parts of the house, were
constant reminders of this problem. While I was there for the interview, he received two phone calls from collection agencies about
medical bills. His retiree health insurance paid only for some, and
he showed me bills for thousands of dollars that he could not pay.
Neither he nor his wife were eligible for the Medicare program yet.
He proudly declared early in the interview, "I didn't owe one dime to
nobody for nothin' before this." And then he shamefully admitted,
"But now even our small savings is used up." He continued, "I used to
be able to do some garage work part-time [car repair work], but I can't
do any garage work now because I have to be here with my wife."

He was at his wits' end and did not know what to do. His wife
was involved in a research program, and was on an experimental

drug for dementia, but the insurance did not cover all the medical visits that were necessary to monitor the effects of the drug. Mr. Martin had not realized this when he started his wife in the program. He admitted:

Every time I go there she needs to see the doctor and that adds $200 onto my bill. I'm looking at a $1,100 bill because my Blue Cross doesn't cover that. I'm suppose to go on Tuesday, but I'm not going to go anymore. It's just not good for me. I just have to get away from those doctor bills.

Throughout the course of our three-hour interview, Mr. Martin kept returning to this pressing issue of his outstanding medical bills and tried to think up ways he could possibly pay them.

Adding to Mr. Martin's stress are recurrent robberies at their home, three times to date during visits to the doctor. These robberies occurred three times in a six-month period, so the insurance company canceled their house insurance. He was finally able to get new insurance, but it initially cost twice as much as his original policy with less coverage.

Their daughter has offered to take care of her mother sometimes on the weekend to give Mr. Martin some relief, but he is reluctant to do this. It's a 70-mile trip to the town where his daughter lives, and he does not like leaving his home now for lengthy periods of time. He also believes that only he can give the proper care to his wife. He is very concerned about his wife's help, but also is very controlling. Talking about the care he provides her, he said:

I give her a bath every other day. I know she eats. During the day she is not going to go hungry. I know she gets her blood pressure pills and eye drops twice a day, whereas in town it might get skipped. My daughter has two little kids and it's hard to take care of my wife.

He paused for a moment and let out a big sigh:

I thought, maybe I should sell this place and move into town. I wish this house was maybe 20 miles closer into the city. But I don't want to. . . . I put the hole in the ground that we put this house in. I took three months off from work. I got six Amish fellows, and we built the house.

I don't want to move back into the city, but I know I am gonna have to do something. I just haven't got it all together. Maybe if I ever get things straightened out. I always thought as long as I had a couple of pennies I could put some gas in the car and have a decent car and jump in it and go, it would be okay, but it made a difference when my wife got sick.

Mr. Martin still has not realistically accepted some of his wife's limitations due to the disease. He still buys complex crossword puzzles and large, complicated jigsaw puzzles, and attempts to interest her in such activities. He gets very frustrated with her when she seems unable or uninterested in those activities she used to like. He even bought her an easel and paint set, because she liked to paint, but she showed no interest in that either. He gets annoyed with her when she cannot sit through a television program, and she constantly gets up and wanders around the house. There is no doubt that some sort of respite care would provide much-needed relief for Mr. Martin and give him some time for himself. He admits, "It was a help when I would be out in my own garage working, but I can't do that now 'cause I spend all my time with her." Yet, when the possibility of using respite services is suggested, it is met with much reluctance, even those services that would be of little or no cost.

Mr. Martin is at a crossroads in his caregiving experience. His wife's condition is worsening, the medical bills are mounting, his isolated home in the country, which once gave him immense pleasure, now seems like a besieged fortress, and he does not know what to do. His children live 70 miles away and are willing to help, but he does not want to ask. All of this has caused undue stress on him, and he is physically feeling the stress of caregiving. Mr. Martin said:

I don't sleep much. I be up just about all night. I'd be in thought all night over what I was gonna do and then I'll get up and my wife doesn't want to get up or she doesn't want to take her bath. I wind up going in there on the couch, lying down 'cause she gives me headaches. I think that's why I have these headaches all the time. I have these tremendous headaches. They can be rough. I got her blood pressure in good shape, but mine . . . that's probably why I have the headaches also. I have to get some sleep or something. I hate for it to get like this.

The one source of support that Mr. Martin has accepted and that seems to provide much needed relief and social outlet is the Alzheimer's Association support group for couples dealing with the early stage of dementia. He referred to this group at least five times throughout the three-hour interview, and it is the only time that his tense body physically relaxed and he smiled. He discussed his experience:

We didn't miss once [the support group was 70 miles away] and believe me, I was a little leery at the time. The support group, I really liked it. I learned a lot. The support group quite naturally gave me a chance to get out of the house, but I learned something every day. I learned from talking to other people. I talked to the people ever since the support group has been over. A couple of the people called me and talked to me. They wanted me to come to a Christmas party. I've read about halfway through the literature. I really got a lot from the support group.

Mr. Martin and Mr. Kerns are "men in transition" caregivers. They are men dealing predominantly with the first level of this change. They are deciding the best course of action to choose as they take on more and more of the caregiving role. In this process, the frustrations and stresses of caregiving are blatantly evident.

"Men in transition" caregivers on the second (psychological) level are struggling more with the psychological impact of their wife's illness on themselves, and the changes in themselves that need to take place at a time in their life when they have little control. The next narrative illustrates this struggle.

Dr. Fifer

As I arrived at Dr. Fifer's home in the retirement community where he and his wife recently moved, he was waiting for me at the door. Dr. Fifer is a dapper, slender 91-year-old retired physician. He was leaning on a cane and wearing a fishing cap, which complemented his attire. Because of his arthritis, he has difficulty walking; he also has some hearing loss and severe vision problems. Although he is struggling to accept his wife's recent diagnosis of Alzheimer's disease, he has great insights into his struggle.

Dr. Fifer immediately started out the interview by discussing two men he is acquainted with who also have wives in various stages of dementia, and how they are coping with it. Dr. Fifer was amazed with one man, a former physician, because of this man's capacity to accept his wife's condition and provide outstanding care to her by himself. In Dr. Fifer's words, "His care was beyond my imagination." The other man, a neighbor at the retirement center, would not believe or accept his wife's behavior. Dr. Fifer said, "He thought she was just misbehaving. She went downhill rather fast." I asked him where he felt he compared on this spectrum of care: "I'm more like the second man in that I cannot accept the changes in her [his wife] until I've had a chance to see that it's the disease. I know of course it is, but I don't want to accept the fact."

He feels that everything is out of his control and that his whole world is being turned upside down. He continued:

This person [his wife] who's been my mainstay, who I consult about everything. I can't do it anymore. She doesn't trust me [anymore]. It's not her fault. The reason she doesn't trust me is she can't trust herself. She doesn't trust herself, so she doesn't trust me. We moved here because we knew we were skating on thin ice, but when it happens, it's—I'M NOT READY.

Mrs. Fifer is still able to do some of the light household chores such as washing, ironing, and putting her clothes away. She is unable to cook anymore because it is too complex and composed of too many steps. Dr. Fifer has had to take on some of the cooking, though they can eat their dinners in the dining room of the retirement center. In his effort to do the household chores, he has set up a system, and when she tries to help him, it upsets his organization.

The other thing is she has always been a helper in anything I start to do, she'd be around to help. She still likes to help. Now, if she helps, she gets it wrong and it spoils my chain of doing things. It interfered with that. It throws me all off and irritates me. I'm am so near the end of my reservoir of strength and I don't know what to expect.

He's found what helps him in this situation is to "take hold of the situation, think about it and realize what's happening. And reason it out."

In discussing the change in their relationship, he said, "You're just a part of her, and if something's wrong,—wham it affects you. We lived together long enough and she could take a look at me and tell how I feel." They still can enjoy each other and close moments at night as they "hug and lay in each other's arms."

Dr. Fifer is a very gregarious person who enjoyed being a physician and talking with his patients and their families. He feels very socially isolated with his wife's disease, and had hoped that moving to a retirement center would offer more people with whom to socialize, but this has not worked out. It seems to him everyone keeps to themselves, although he related an incident that occurred the day before that gave him much pleasure:

It's good for me to have a break and get out with normal people. It's good for me. For instance, yesterday I had a problem with my toaster, so I took it over to the gang that takes care of maintenance [because of his arthritis and limited vision, he uses a golf cart to go around the complex]. I know a couple of the boys pretty good, and they were having lunch and they gave me some hot sauce and potato chips and we kidded around. We had a great time, and that was good for me. I need to talk to somebody for a little while or something like that.

Dr. Fifer has been able to find a confidant in one of his daughters who lives nearby. He can truly express and confide his feelings to her, which provides much comfort and relief for him. He has grown closer to his daughter since his wife's illness, and this is a source of great joy for him.

When asked for advice he would give to other husbands caring for a wife with dementia, he had these thoughts:

I guess the important thing is to accept these changes as the disease and accept the irritating behavior as part of the disease. The men of our generation have been used to being in charge, and they are not used to being wrong or not knowing what to do.

Conclusions
The 30 husbands in this study adjusted in diverse ways to their new caregiving role. Some used a "work" orientation, and this helped

them to cope with their wives' illness and restore some order into their rapidly changing world. Some found that their love for their wives sustained them and provided meaning, sustenance, and motivation for the tasks ahead. Yet for some of the husbands, their marital vows, loyalty, and sense of responsibility spurred them to shoulder the obligations of caring for a wife with dementia. For some husbands with their wives in the early stage of the disease, a team approach was still possible; as a couple, they could make some plans together. And finally, there were the men who were transitioning their identities to caregiver and struggling with the demands of that change. They were men in transition, and this transition caused much frustration, anger, and caregiver stress.

There are a number of questions that need to be asked about this proposed typology of husband caregivers. For one, are the types mutually exclusive? For example, could a husband who oriented to his caregiver role out of a sense of duty also feel much love and compassion for his wife? Yes, of course, but that was not the overriding pattern of experience that emerged from the interviews. Another question is, do these orientations to caregiving change over time or are they constant? This study can not fully answer that question, since it was a cross-sectional study that looked at a group of men at one period in their caregiving experiences. There is no doubt that two of the categories would have to change, "going it together" and "men in transition." As the wife's illness progressed, working together as husband and wife would no longer be possible; the men who are in transition or at the crossroads would probably transition to one of the other categories. As for the three other types, their way of adjusting might seem stable, but it is difficult to predict.

What we have tried to present to you, as is indicated by the title of this chapter ("toward" a typology of husband caregivers), is a typology that still may be in process. More research on male caregivers is needed to verify or dispute these findings.

Chapter Four
Husbands
Service Implications—What Can We Learn?

Until recently, people who care for those suffering from Alzheimer's disease and related disorders typically had a limited number of resources and services available to them. In response to the increasing number of individuals with the disease and their caregivers, medical advancements in early diagnosis, greater public awareness, and a growing network of Alzheimer's Association chapters and other health and social service agencies focusing on dementia, there now exists an expanding range of programs geared to the needs of Alzheimer's patients and their caregivers. Some types of services that are available are information and referral, educational programs, literature on Alzheimer's disease, support groups, case management, adult day care, respite services, homemaker and personal care services (many of which are discussed below). Most of these services, though, are offered on a fee-for-service basis and availability of these services is often limited outside a large urban area.

As indicated in Appendix B (Table 1), many of the husbands were using some of the services mentioned above, which they found to be a beneficial supplemental support in their efforts to provide care to their wives. These husbands, as well as those who had not used any services, voiced suggestions during the interviews for the development of new services they thought would particularly meet their needs as caregivers. Their suggestions included gender-specific services as well as programs and services that cut across gender lines and could be helpful to all caregivers.

This chapter provides a summary of these recommended services. The husbands' suggestions are divided into three main areas: social support programs, educational programs, and respite and other related services and supports.

Our sample of husband caregivers is small and nonrandom, so generalization of their needs to other populations of husband caregivers is limited. However, we offer these recommendations in the hope that they will stimulate a dialogue among service providers to consider the specific service needs of the male caregiver population with which they are working. We hope this dialogue will ultimately result in increased implementation of programs and services to meet the ever-growing needs of male caregivers.

Social Support Programs

Social support programs discussed by the husbands covered three areas: (1) traditional support groups; (2) specialized support groups, such as all male, early diagnosed, and computer networks, and (3) social networking activities/opportunities. Because so much has already been written on traditional support groups (Toseland and Rossiter, 1989), we focus on the other two major areas of recommendations.

Support Groups

Support groups in general provide three types of assistance to caregivers. They provide *emotional support* and serve as a network for establishing friendships. They are a source of *accurate up-to-date information* on dementia. In addition, they also provide the caregiver with *how-to tips on day-to-day care management* (Montgomery, 1995).

Although most husbands in our study expressed the need for more social support, many of the men we interviewed responded that they were hesitant about attending a support group. It was one of the services they initially thought they didn't need and going to a group was often done only because a friend or relative insisted that they attend a session.

Once they had attended a group session, we found their reactions depended on the type and makeup of the group and where the husband was in the caregiving process; that is, whether he was caring for a wife in the early, middle, or late stage of dementia. Some husbands preferred groups composed of all men, rather than mixed-gender groups. Some husbands caring for a wife in the early stage of dementia were overwhelmed and depressed by the issues raised by caregivers caring for a relative in the later stage of the disease. Other husbands felt uncomfortable with the psychosocial support group format. The types of support groups that husbands found helpful were the all-male support group, the early stage support program, and the computer networks.

Male Support Groups

Many men felt uncomfortable attending traditional support groups that were composed primarily of female caregivers. They felt uncomfortable talking about emotional and sensitive issues such as sexuality and dating. They were embarrassed about baring their souls in front of women caregivers. Those men that had the opportunity to attend an all-male support group felt freedom to express their range of emotions and reported a special camaraderie among the participants that had not developed among more traditional support groups.

There are many models of male support groups (Kaye and Applegate, 1990a). Husbands in this study identified critical features in the structure and format of such a group. These critical features were a male facilitator, a facilitator with a nursing background (to provide a resource on medical and personal care issues), and a nonjudgmental atmosphere that allowed for open discussion of sensitive issues. Most important is that this type of group provide a level of comfort and trust where the men feel safe in sharing their thoughts and feelings. Perhaps, as these men become more accepting of their caregiving role and more at ease in sharing their feelings and thoughts, they may be more willing to participate in the traditional mixed-gender support groups.

Most of the men who brought up the need for male support groups fell into the categories of "labor of love" and "men in transition." The "labor of love" husbands needed a safe place where they could discuss their sadness and feelings about the change in their relationship and the loss of their loved one. The "men in transition" husbands wanted to discuss their transition into a caregiving role with other men who were in similar situations.

Early Stage Support Programs

Some of the men reported that many of the support groups they were referred to included caregivers who oftentimes were in the later stage of caring for a relative with Alzheimer's disease. Hearing about the end stage of the disease, including problems with nursing home care, overwhelmed husbands whose wives were in the early to middle stages of the disease. This was especially true when the husbands themselves were still adjusting to their role as caregiver. These husbands, after a first visit, were reluctant to return to the support group.

Several of the men in our study had participated in a specialized support group for people in the early stage of the disease and their families. In this model program, the person with the illness has to be aware of their diagnosis and able to participate in group discussions. The person with the illness must attend with at least one other family member. Members meet weekly for two-hour sessions over eight weeks. A maximum of eight family units are invited to participate in these series. The sessions, facilitated by two clinically trained social work professionals and assisted by a volunteer who has past caregiving experience, focus on information about the disease and coping strategies for couples and other family members. Session topics include an overview of Alzheimer's disease, current research, memory-enhancing techniques, how to work together with your family as a team, communication, giving and getting support, how to cope, and local resources available. Breakout sessions are an integral part of the format that allows time for people with the illness to meet together separately from the caregivers so that each group can discuss their unique issues. Reuniting at the end of these breakout sessions sometimes encourages couples to discuss with each other difficult issues that they had previously avoided, such as driving, sexual relations, and overprotectiveness, among others. The entire focus of the program is on team building and helping family units plan together for the future (see Appendix C).

This program's focus on the person with the disease took away some of the reluctance that husbands had in attending more traditional support groups: The group wasn't *just* for them; it was also for their wives.

This type of program seemed particularly helpful to those husbands who were typed as "going it together" and "men in transition." The "going it together" husbands who had attended this type of support group truly appreciated the team approach of the program. Information about the disease was given to these couples together, and they were encouraged to make decisions jointly that fit their whole approach to caregiving. For the "men in transition" husbands, the program allowed the familiarity of old roles, as they were able to attend as a couple and socially interact with other couples. Because the program was made up of people who were all in the early stage of caregiving, it provided a safe place where these "men in transition" husbands could express their feelings about the confusion, changes, and dilemmas they were experiencing, even overcoming their discomfort about disclosing their feelings in a mixed-gender group. It also helped them learn new skills and start to perceive themselves as caregivers.

Husbands who found traditional support groups initially overwhelming discovered that this structured program, which included the person with memory loss, was a more comfortable way of talking about the realities of caregiving and Alzheimer's disease. Many of these men kept contact with group members long after the scheduled sessions ended.

Computer Support Networks
Another method of support in which some of the men in our study participated, and from which they obtained great comfort and reassurance, was a computer support network designed for Alzheimer's caregivers. This interactive telecomputing system could be accessed if the caregiver had a computer and a modem (a device that allows one computer to "talk" to another computer over the telephone lines). By dialing into a system called Free-Net, caregivers could leave messages and "talk" to other caregivers without ever leaving their homes (Smyth and Harris, 1993).

This system not only had the features of other support groups mentioned above, but it also had special features, unique to this medium, to which many husbands could particularly relate. Caregivers were able to access Free-Net any time of the day or night. Thus, a caregiver could get support whenever he felt the need, be it noon or midnight. The system also allowed participants to remain anonymous, if they so chose. You did not need to give your name or any identifying information. So men, who often have difficulty expressing their thoughts and feelings to others, did not have to reveal who was "talking."

Use of the computer also affords a caregiver a sense of control, an important issue for men. One can enter into a discussion as one wishes, reveal as much or as little as one likes, or just be an observer to the discussions of others (unless you type something on the screen, no one knows you are there). The men have control over the level of their involvement. The timing and use of the service is also totally in the control of the user. In addition, using a computer adds a technical, scientific dimension to the caregiving process, which appealed to many of the men (see Appendix D).

The attraction of this type of support tool is growing, and many communities throughout the United States are developing their own telecomputing systems. From our limited sample, this computer support network seemed to appeal particularly to two groups of husband caregivers, the "men in transition" and "the workers." For the "men in transition," as their needs were changing on almost a day-to-day basis, the computer seemed to provide them with the ready 24-hour-a-day support and up-to-date information that they needed. "The worker" husbands were often already familiar with computers and used the system to obtain accurate information on dementia from computer bulletin boards at any time of the day or night. They were not as likely to use computers for emotional support.

These specialized support groups—the all-male group, the early diagnosed group, and the computer support network—show great promise for ongoing support for male caregivers. The latter two would be beneficial for women caregivers as well.

Social Networking Activities

From our discussions with the husband caregivers, social networking activities were recommended as a high priority to deal with their increasing feelings of social isolation. In particular, what was recommended was the development of friendship clubs, with the focus being a common hobby or interest.

Friendship Clubs

Sometimes the strongest need voiced by the men in the study was for support of a more informal nature. As is reported by many caregivers, friends and supports distanced themselves once the Alzheimer's disease diagnosis was known. Many of the husbands in our study were very lonely. This was especially true of those men who fell into the "labor of love" group. These men had lost their companions and closest friends, and they expressed the greatest degree of social isolation. They had depended on their wives for their social support and networking. With their wives no longer able to function in this capacity, their friendship circles fell apart.

What many of these men were missing was a supportive peer group, someplace where they could just relax and take a break from caregiving; as one caregiver stated, "to run away" from their caregiving duties. They also needed something that linked them back to their former lives and self-identities.

Friendship groups or clubs based upon shared hobbies or interests would serve to meet the needs of these men who lacked peer support. These groups could revolve around hobbies such as fishing, golfing, or biking (hobbies that many of the male caregivers in this study shared). These clubs could easily spin off from other caregiver support groups or could be formed independently.

The important feature here is that the men have control over the content and structure of these clubs and, once started, these clubs should not be professionally facilitated. A benefit to forming these types of clubs with other caregivers is that there is an understanding among members about the burdens and demands that may keep the caregiver from fully participating in their hobby, as well as consistently attending these meetings. These clubs could meet periodically, go on outings (with respite care arranged for their wives), and fill in the social supports that are missing for many male caregivers. This type of program would be of greatest benefit to the "labor of love" and "sense of duty" caregivers.

Social support programs, whether they are traditional support groups, specialized support groups or social networking activities, can provide the male caregiver with much needed encouragement and a sense of belonging and connectedness with others.

Educational Programs

Husbands wanted more education and information about the disease and about caregiving. They also suggested that other groups and individuals that they interacted with needed more information about dementia and the strains of caregiving. Based on their recommendations, in this section we discuss the need for specific types of educational programs. These programs fall under three categories: caregiver education, professional education, and education for friends and colleagues.

Caregiver Education

Many of the men in our study took advantage of programs and workshops about Alzheimer's disease offered in the community. Those who attended these classes said they found them helpful. The classes provided them with a better understanding of the disease and a better understanding of their wives' behavior. What they particularly felt they needed was training in personal care skills, cooking, financial management, and how to hire help. As one might expect of men who were raised in the 1920s and 1930s, they were often ill equipped to take on the chores of cooking, household management, and caring for the personal needs of an ill wife.

Personal Care Classes

We recommend that agencies serving male caregivers hold classes periodically whose primary focus is teaching personal care skills. Classes should focus on how to bathe an adult female, with emphasis on safety in the bathroom, toileting, female hygiene, and grooming.

Tips and shortcuts on how to dress a woman would be very helpful to many of the husbands. Those men in our study who were in the early stage of caring for their wives were trying to help their wives maintain their predisease routines. Many of these men were struggling with helping their wives put on stockings and apply makeup. Men dealing with the later stage of dementia were more focused on function over appearance in regard to dressing. Men at this stage found it helpful to use elastic waist pants and Velcro fasteners rather than dresses with zippers and stockings. All these men need a safe place to discuss and learn the "how to's" of these tasks.

Cooking Classes

For many of the husbands, cooking was not a well-developed skill and one they approached with much trepidation. Cooking also had an emotional component, which was discussed earlier (see Chapter 2). These men needed information not only on how to cook for their wives but also on how to satisfy their own nutritional needs. Most helpful would be basic cooking classes that include tips on nutrition, feeding techniques, and recipes geared towards the ethnic and cultural tastes of these men.

Financial and Household Management Classes

Another series of classes that is needed for husband caregivers is on financial and household management. The men in our study were split on how they handled the finances in their relationships prior to the onset of the illness: Some of the men were in charge of bill paying and finances, while others basically handed over their paychecks to their wives. Caregivers who have never had the financial responsibility of running the home often found this an additional stress to their many other duties.

An area of financial management that was particularly stressful for many husbands involved the handling of medical bills and insurance. A number of the men interviewed had shoe boxes filled with overdue medical bills and insurance forms stacked on kitchen tables or scattered around their homes. An instructional class that focuses on household management and addresses the issues of check writing and checkbook balancing, how to submit insurance claims, and budgeting would be beneficial to many husbands.

Hiring Help

Another specific training module recommended that would help these husbands is instruction on how to hire, train, and best use respite and chore workers. Many of the men in the middle and later stages of caregiving were ready to hire help but didn't know where to go, whom to hire or what questions to ask. This training program should include the various types of service available in the community (explaining the difference between personal care, chore services, respite, etc.), how to get help through an agency or privately, sample interview questions, a sample contract, what a caregiver should expect from the worker, and how to be a partner with the hired caregiver (see Appendix E).

Some of the caregivers expressed a need for an employment service that specifically trains workers to care for people with dementia. They wanted this service to be affordable and without arbitrary hourly minimums that often restricted flexibility in hiring workers when they needed them.

All these classes would address the needs across all the types of husbands described in Chapter 3 but particularly would be helpful to the "men in transition" husbands who were in a state of crisis. These men were coping with their changed roles, sorting out their emotions, and trying to gain some control over their lives. Men whose caregiving roles had not changed for awhile had for the most part mastered many of these household skills (or hired someone else to perform them) and were more concerned with dealing with the behavioral changes or secondary illnesses associated with the disease.

Professional Education

Almost across the board, the men in this study voiced strong service suggestions for the various professionals they encountered, particularly health care professionals such as doctors, nurses, and social workers, as well as clergy. Recommended education for health care professionals included issues relating to diagnosis, the caregiver in the care plan, and awareness of the psychological needs of the caregiver.

Recommendations for Health Care Professionals

Diagnosis. As stated earlier, many of these men were terribly frustrated at the time of diagnosis. They were left with ambiguous information from their doctors. Almost unanimously, the husbands studied here said it would have been helpful to them to be told directly of the diagnosis (or the suspected diagnosis). Having a better understanding of what they were dealing with would have helped them in planning and coping with their wives' illness. Clear information along with a direct referral to a helping organization such as the Alzheimer's Association would have assisted these men in getting help sooner. These men wanted to obtain information in a manner that did not overwhelm and eliminate all hope.

Physicians and social workers need to be educated about the needs of these caregivers so they are aware of how best to assist these men. Diagnosis is a critical time when husbands can be linked immediately to other helping professionals and services. If their experience is poor at this stage, they may be more reluctant to ask for help later on.

Care Plan. Another frustration for these men was that they felt like outsiders to the health care team. They did not feel they were included in the discussions and care planning for their wives. Even when present at team meetings they felt their input was not listened to or valued. They wanted to be an integral part of their wives' health care teams. All team members need to understand the role of the spouse caregivers and integrate them into their team approach.

Psychological Needs. Some of the complex psychological issues these men deal with are depression and suicide ideation. Health care professionals need to be alert to signs of caregiver depression. In only rare instances were caregivers getting treatment for these problems. It is recommended that health care professionals assess the needs of the caregiver as well as the person with Alzheimer's when they have contact with these couples. Older men have very high rates of suicide compared to the general population (Osgood, 1985).

Recommendations for Clergy
In times of crisis, religious leaders are often the first people these men turn to for support and comfort. It is important that the clergy have accurate, up-to-date knowledge and information about Alzheimer's. Sometimes religious institutions were well prepared to provide the necessary help, including support groups, respite programs, and so on. Others were not able to meet the needs of these caregivers. Ongoing education about dementia needs to be available to pastoral care professionals and clergy of all denominations. Educational programs and literature about the disease should be available to congregants as well.

Education for Friends and Colleagues
We often heard from these men how devastated they were when their friends deserted them after the diagnosis. Many of the men realized that people had misconceptions about the disease and didn't know how to be helpful. For husbands who are still working or recently retired, colleagues and supervisors often had no understanding of how they could best be supportive.

A brochure specifically oriented to friends and colleagues that educates them about the basics of dementia, confronts misconceptions, and gives tips on how to be most helpful to caregivers and the family member with dementia would fill this need.

Also for husbands still in the work force, retirement-planning programs that include information on Alzheimer's disease would help alleviate misconceptions and provide a basis for understanding the issues that male caregivers (as well as female caregivers in the work force) face. Employee Assistance Program (EAP) counselors should have some awareness of the issues surrounding the care of a relative with dementia, as well as available educational literature and knowledge about community resources.

Educational programs, be they for caregivers, health care providers, friends, or the public, are a vital source of support for husbands caring for wives with dementia. Innovative educational programs need to be developed that truly meet the special multiple needs of men taking on the caregiving role.

Respite and Other Related Services and Supports

Respite for the men who were long-term caregivers was the critical factor that allowed them to continue caring for their wives at home. As many husbands said, it was that time away with activities for themselves that gave them the rest and strength they needed to continue. Many men caring for a wife in the early and middle stages of dementia were in the process of trying to obtain some respite care to aid them in the caregiving process. "Respite" is a broad term that covers many different types of services that provide time away, or breaks, in the caregiving routine. Respite services can include in-home care, adult day care programs, and weekend or vacation care. Respite can be provided by family members—children, siblings, cousins—but for consistent services, most of the men felt the need to rely on paid care providers.

Respite

Across the 30 husbands interviewed, multiple types of paid respite care were used. For some husbands, respite meant using a nearby adult day care program three days a week. For other husbands, what was helpful for them was a companion for their wife in their home for a set number of hours a week. Other husbands would occasionally go away on vacation for a week and place their wife in a short-term stay bed of a nursing home. Each man used the type of respite that best met his needs and ability to pay.

A critical feature of any of the respite programs for the husbands was that it had to be flexible, able to meet the hours and days that would best meet their specific needs. The respite programs also had to be affordable, as there were limited outside funds for such relief. A few of the husbands could have desperately used some consistent structured relief, but due to cost could not obtain the services. Husbands had to feel their wives would be receiving good quality care. A number of husbands cut their vacations short when they thought their wives were not receiving satisfactory care.

Other Services and Supports
Public Restrooms and Travel Companions
Many of the men who had retired reported great joy in traveling with their wives. As the disease progressed, they felt they had to cut back on these trips and grieved for the ability to even take long drives together. Several of these men reported that the biggest factor restricting them from traveling with their wives was toileting. As their wives needed more supervision, they could no longer be trusted to go into the ladies' room on their own. The problem is with public restrooms: Societal norms do not allow men to accompany their wives into public restrooms, nor does it allow the women to go with their husbands into the men's room. This was a dilemma that none of the husbands in our study was able to overcome, and many couples were restricted to taking only short trips away from home. These restrictions would be lifted if rest stops and restaurants provided at least one single-stall unisex toilet. This way a husband could escort his wife into the bathroom without causing a scene or taking the risk of letting her go by herself.

Another solution to this problem would be for the husbands to hire a travel companion. This would be a female who would be willing to accompany these couples on their trips. This person would not only assist with toileting, but would be an extra set of eyes and hands to help out and supervise the person with Alzheimer's, giving relief to the caregiver and allowing another type of respite to take place.

Volunteer and Advocacy Opportunities
A number of the husbands in the study used their free time, pro-

vided by respite services, to become active volunteers for Alzheimer's-related causes. The men stated they volunteered for two main reasons: altruism and giving back to the cause. As they became involved volunteers, they also developed new friendships and expanded their social networks.

The men from our research who shared the characteristics of the "sense of duty" group were most often the volunteers. They made good candidates for volunteers because of their strong sense of duty and responsibility. They received satisfaction from contributing back to others by way of volunteer activities as community speakers, support group leaders, political advocates, research participants, and so on. They reported feeling useful and empowered through their involvement. Through these activities their social networks increased and their networks expanded. Social workers and health care professionals should not overlook the multiple benefits of volunteering for the male caregiver (Harris, 1995).

Conclusion

It is clear from the husbands studied that programs offered to caregivers must be expanded and specialized if providers want to meet the needs of male caregivers. As services are added it is likely that agencies will attract many previously unserved husband caregivers. As more services for male caregivers develop, service providers familiar with the husband typologies described in Chapter 3 can link husband caregivers with the services they are most likely to use and from which they can gain the greatest benefit. Service professionals may use Table 4.1 (at the end of this chapter) as a guide to consider evaluating what program might be beneficial for a particular husband caregiver.

Many of our recommendations can be implemented by agencies that are already providing caregiver services. For example, adding an all-male support group or an early diagnosed group will not be a major change of course for a provider who is already offering traditional support group programs. Agencies that provide caregiver education can add seminars on cooking, personal hygiene, or financial management. Targeting education on Alzheimer's to professionals and the general public needs to be expanded to include the specific topics and issues mentioned earlier.

Some recommendations may lead to new programs. Developing a dementia-specific computer bulletin board can be a rewarding (and potentially grant fundable) project that can be linked into the multitude of computer networks that are currently available in many communities. Friendship clubs can be initiated by any number of agencies such as the Alzheimer's Association, senior centers, and churches. Once initiated, the agency may need act only as the host site.

Other recommendations, such as flexible and affordable respite, or unisex toilets, may require resources beyond what a single agency has available. These changes will involve a high level of commitment and innovative problem solving to implement.

There is a particular poignancy to the problems faced by these caregiving husbands. Each in his own unique fashion has made a commitment to caring for his spouse at extreme personal sacrifice. The community at large has not yet acknowledged the special needs of male caregivers. Thus, the husbands in our study often felt they were facing this monumental task alone. Their insights expose the gaps in the current service-delivery system and serve as a challenge to the professional community to recognize and meet their needs.

Table 4:1 Husband Caregivers Service and Program Summary

The following is a summarized version of the suggested services and programs discussed in Chapter 4 linked to the type of husband caregiver most likely to utilize or benefit from those services. These indications are generalizations, and clearly not every caregiver in each typology would find these programs helpful, nor should a caregiver be excluded from a program because of his typology. This chart should function solely as a guide to human service professionals in linking husband caregivers to services.

	Typology				
	The Worker	Labor of Love	Sense of Duty	Going It Together	Men in Transition
Service					
Male Support Group		x			x
Early Stage Group				x	x
Computer Support Networks	x				x
Friendship Clubs		x	x		
Caregiver Education	x	x	x	x	x
Respite	x	x	x	x	x
Volunteer Programs			x		

Part Two

Sons as Caregivers

Their Inner World

Chapter Five
Sons' Characteristics, Common Themes, and Shared Experiences

The 30 sons interviewed played a major role in caring for a parent with dementia. The most common cause of this dementia was Alzheimer's disease. The caregiving tasks in which the sons were involved varied depending on the family situations and needs of the ill parent. Some sons were providing hands-on personal care to mothers and fathers that included chores such as bathing, dressing, cooking, and feeding. Other sons' roles, often when there was a healthy parent providing the hands-on care to the other ill parent, were that of helping to "care for the caregiver." These sons provided such tasks as emotional support, respite care, financial advice, transportation, and information-seeking and patient-advocacy functions. Some sons provided all caregiving tasks, and some sons shared responsibilities with siblings. All of the sons were involved in the decision-making process for their parents, and many took leadership roles.

The quality of the relationships with their parents over the years varied. Some sons had relationships that were warm and close, others had cold and distant relationships, and still others had volatile ones. But regardless of the past relationship, the filial ties were strong and all the sons interviewed were committed to care for their parents.

This chapter focuses on these sons by first presenting a demographic profile that describes characteristics of this son sample, factors such as their educational, occupational, and religious backgrounds, as well as sibling information. Some of this information is examined in light of the influence it might have on sons' motivation for caregiving. The second part of the chapter delves deeper, probing into the thoughts and feelings of the sons, their inner worlds, as they struggled to care for a parent with dementia.

Characteristics of the Sons

The 30 sons were mostly college graduates; only 27 percent of the sample did not have a college degree (see Appendix B, Table 2). As reflected by their educational level, only 7 percent of the sample had incomes $10,000 or under, and 40 percent had incomes over $60,000 a year. It was predominantly a middle-class sample, with much variation within that group. Their occupations were quite diverse: construction workers, factory workers, postmen, teachers, artists, salesmen, business executives, entrepreneurs, and college professors. One son was unemployed and on disability leave; 23 percent of the sons were retired.

Their average age was 50 years old. They ranged from a 32-year-old stockbroker who has been caring for his mother with Alzheimer's disease at home for 10 years, to a 71-year-old semiretired real estate agent whose 96-year-old mother had just entered a nursing home after a major stroke. The majority of the sons were married, but a significant portion, 40 percent of the sons in the study, were either never married, widowed, or divorced. Seventeen percent of the sample was African-American.

Interestingly, over 50 percent of the sons who volunteered to participate in this study were Catholic, which is notably higher than the 30 percent of the population that is Catholic in the Cleveland area or the 21 percent nationally. Religious affiliation is not a factor that is often closely examined in caregiving studies and is just beginning to be scrutinized (McFadden, 1994).

A number of factors have been proposed by researchers as potentially having an impact on a son's involvement in caregiving to an ill parent, and some of the demographic information presented below is discussed in this light. Some factors suggested are gender issues, particularly the availability of a sister (Brody, 1989, 1990), geographic proximity (Finley, Roberts, and Banahan, 1988), and sex of the parent (Lee, Dwyer, and Coward, 1993).

Seventy-seven percent of the sons in the study had siblings, with the majority of the sons having sisters, 43 percent of whom lived in town. Since it is usually assumed that a daughter will provide the care to an ill parent, there appeared to be factors other than the unavailability of sisters that influenced this sample of sons to provide care to their parents.

It is also usually assumed that the child who is geographically closest to the parent will be more involved in his/her parent's care. In this sample, 50 percent of the sons were the only sibling in the same town as their parents, but 8 of these 15 sons had moved their parents to the Cleveland area to be near them. So, it was not the convenience of the geographic proximity of the parent that was an influencing factor for this sample of sons. An additional finding, which questions the influence of geographic proximity on these sons' motivation for caregiving, was that 50 percent of the sample had other siblings living in town, yet these sons were the active caregivers.

In examining the influence of the sex of the ill parent on the sons' involvement in caregiving, again from just demographic information, this factor does not appear to be a strong influence. The assumption is that sons will be more comfortable providing care, especially hands-on care, to their fathers than to their mothers. Sons in this study, though, were involved in caring for both fathers and mothers (33 percent and 67 percent, respectively), which is equal to the proportion nationally of men and women over the age of 65 in the United States. Thus, the sex of the parent did not seem to be a relevant factor.

Sibling birth order is another variable often discussed as relevant to sons' involvement in caregiving. It is an expectation in some families that if a son is involved in caring for a parent, the oldest son will assume that responsibility. Yet in this sample of son caregivers, only 17 percent of the caregivers were the oldest sibling. Thus, birth order overall did not seem to have a major impact on a son's motivation to become involved in caring for his parent with dementia.

Therefore, demographic and family structural variables such as availability of a sister, geographic proximity, sex of parent, and birth order appeared to have limited influence on these sons' decisions to become involved in caring for a parent with dementia.

The average age of the parent with dementia was 77 years old with a range of 63 to 96 years. Although the parent tended to be in the early and middle stages of the disease process, almost one-quarter of the sample lived in nursing homes. Other research has shown that children are more likely to place a parent in a nursing home than a spouse. Spouses will go beyond their limits of caregiving for a longer period of time than adult children (Johnson, 1983). However, it should also be noted that almost one-quarter of this sample of sons had their parents living with them.

The two formal support services that sons most often used were a telephone helpline for information and referral, and educational literature on Alzheimer's disease; over 70 percent of the sample used these two services. Sons were most often the initial information gatherers for the family. It was a pivotal role they played.

To conclude, the sons in this study were predominantly middle class from various occupations, but they did not easily fit the usual assumptions made about son caregivers. Many were involved in caring for a parent, even though they had sisters. The geographic proximity of a parent did not appear to act as a key detriment or impetus in their involvement, nor did the sex of the parent, as sons were as involved with mothers as with fathers. These sons were as likely to have a parent living in a nursing home as in their own home, and the key services they accessed were information/referral and educational services. By focusing only on sons and not comparing them with daughters, this study has identified more variations in son caregiving than expected.

The common experiences of these son caregivers are introduced below, but first there are three meaningful differences in the interviewing process between sons and husbands that need to be addressed. These observations add to the understanding we seek about male caregivers. Interviewing the sons was qualitatively different from interviewing the husbands for three main reasons.

First, the locations in which the majority of the sons chose to be interviewed were different. It appeared that the sons had more freedom of movement. Many were not involved in the 24-hour care of a relative, and thus they could meet anywhere for the interview. Only five sons chose to meet in their homes. The others requested that the meetings be held in their offices, the researcher's university office, a public library, or a restaurant. These settings were neutral and businesslike, and the sons seemed more comfortable structuring the environment for the interviews in this manner.

Second, there was less emotional intensity in the son's interviews than in the husbands'. This is not to say that the sons lacked emotional involvement in caring for their parents, but the degree and strength of emotions expressed overall was less. The possible reasons for this will be discussed in Chapter 8 in the section on contrasts.

Last, many of the sons described the caregiving process in terms of sport and car analogies. Cars and sports are an integral part of this generation of men's development, and by placing the caregiving into terms with which they can identify, it helped them to make sense of the experience. This made the experience concrete, something with which they were familiar and to which they could relate.

For example, one son used basketball terms to describe handling difficult situations with his father. He said, "The things we thought would be slam dunks [easy to handle] weren't, and things we thought would be difficult were slam dunks." Another son used a car analogy as a way of trying to understand the care an older person needs. He commented, "When you are taking care of an older person, it is a very complex thing. Kind of like a new car with all the special carburetors and injection systems. It's almost as if you do have to go to the computer at some point to identify where the problem might be."

These observations about the meeting places, the emotional intensity of the interviews, and the car and sport analogies describe aspects of son caregiving, to give a flavor of some of the differences in the interviewing process compared to husbands. These help to set the background against which the common themes discussed below can be better understood.

Common Themes and Shared Experiences

The 30 sons, like the husbands, discussed certain themes that appeared again and again in their narratives. Themes evident were duty; acceptance; taking charge; emotions of love, anger, resentment, sadness, and guilt; loss; dealing with siblings; work flexibility; reversing roles; coping strategies; and positive aspects of caregiving. These themes are examined so the reader can gain a deeper understanding of what it is like for a son to take on a caregiving role for an ill parent.

Duty

The most common theme among the 30 sons was their sense of duty to care for their ill parent; their sense of filial obligation was paramount in the interviews. Many sons echoed almost the same words, saying, "You got to do what you got to do." Other sons expressed similar feelings, but with variations.

One 53-year-old son caring for a father in the early stage of dementia, whom he had just moved from Florida into his own home, said matter-of-factly, "It's my responsibility, that's all. So I'm the one to do it." A 46-year-old son expressed to us his thoughts about caring for his 76-year-old mother, who had been ill for many years, even before the dementia:

I guess I might say blood is thicker than water. I don't know if I particularly ever loved my mother, but I have this moral commitment, familial commitment, to take care of her and make sure she is taken care of.

An African-American son talked about a promise he had made to his mother many years ago.

As a kid of four years old, I made a commitment to her that I would always take care of her and I thought when I started hearing about all her weird behavior from family and neighbors [his mother lived out of town] that, "Oh, the Lord's gonna get me now." So I just jumped in the car and went down and got her. I got a grave responsibility.

But perhaps it was a 60-year-old son, whose mother died a few years ago, who said it most poignantly:

What kept me going was my devotion to her. I saw how they [his parents] treated me over my lifetime, the loyalty they felt. I learned. I learned that that's what you do with family. You don't moan and groan about them; you take care of them. You do what you have to do.

Acceptance

These sons for the most part were much more able to accept the diagnosis of dementia in their parent more readily and at an earlier stage in the illness than other family members. This did not mean that they were not upset by the diagnosis, or did not at first attempt to deny the facts; however, when confronted with the conclusion, they accepted the reality and started to make plans. They often set limits for themselves regarding the point at which they would no longer continue to provide the care to their parent. Early in the caregiving process many began to discuss the possibility of having to use a nursing home.

One African-American son, who cared for his mother at home until her death a year ago, expressed his acceptance this way:

You can look at your mother and you can look at the disease, they're entirely different. You remember how sweet and how compassionate your mom was, and you look at the disease over here and it's totally out of character, so you have to try to find a balance. You might as well come out of this denial you're in and recognize the fact that she has a serious problem and begin to help her and yourself by dealing with it.

One son was sharing the responsibility of caring for his father with his brother. His father had been diagnosed three years before and was moving into the middle stage of dementia. The son stated matter-of-factly:

The handwriting on the wall was very plain to see and we needed to do something. We [his brother and himself] went on what I call a 2–3–2 kick. We had brought in a lady to care for our father during the day, but we were staying with him at night and on the weekends. We were trying to split our weekends so that we didn't have to stay with him all day Saturday and all day Sunday. So, whoever would be there Friday night and all day Saturday would be relieved by the other one Sunday morning. And that other person would be there Tuesday, Wednesday, Thursday night, and we'd go home Friday, Saturday [hence 2–3–2]. It was a whole routine that got to be a little bit too much. I think maybe both of us are at the point where we're saying we can't continue in this scheme of things long-term. We are very concerned, but we can't continue to be with him 24 hours a day. We have started to look at nursing homes with special Alzheimer's disease units.

Each son accepted his parent's illness in a different way and expressed it uniquely, but it was this acceptance that let him move on to deal with the issues of caregiving. This "moving on" sometimes resulted in them "taking charge" of the situation and becoming the decision makers.

"Taking Charge"

One of the major roles that many of the sons played in their family was, as they said, "to take charge" of the situation and push the family to make the necessary decisions. It was a theme that was reiterated over and over again in the interviews. This was a role many of the sons felt comfortable with from their world of work and often from their role of being a male in American society. This "taking charge" took various forms.

A 55-year-old son returned home to Cleveland to assume the responsibility of caring for his mother. His sister had their parents living with her, and when her father died and her mother's dementia became worse, he came home to help her. There were other siblings living locally, but he was not married and his occupation allowed him flexibility. Reflecting on his role, he said:

There always seems to be a family captain in a situation like this and no one else was doing it. I was a vice president and used to doing things, getting them done, so I just did it. Called a family meeting. I said if you want me to take responsibility, fine. But, if I am in charge, I am in charge. I formed a task force and we went to look at 15 nursing homes in the area.

One 40-year-old son helped his mother, who was providing more of the hands-on care and wanted her husband to remain at home. The son shouldered the responsibilities for decisions that would be very traumatic for his father. For example, he made the decision about his father's driving.

I told him he could not drive. And then he hated me. I was the root of all his problems. I was his scapegoat for years and years and years. I played the role of the bad guy. And honestly, as far as pinpointing a son's role in things, that's an excellent one.

Another son talked about making the decision that it was time for his father to move to a nursing home.

I was willing to bite the bullet and say, "Look, this is what you got to do. You may be very unhappy with me for making the decision and you may

hate me for it, or at least you may think you hate me for it, but I'm
willing to accept it."

One 71-year-old African-American son, referring to his 96-year-
old mother's move to his house, plainly stated:

I just insisted this is what we have to do. You know, sometimes your
parents get so old and sick that someone has to take charge and make
decisions. Now, if only you can make them in a way that won't antago-
nize them too much.

Many of the sons viewed taking charge of the situation as a natural
extension of the role of a son. However, one of the most frustrating
aspects of trying to "take charge" of this disease, as voiced by a number of sons was, "There were no good answers."

Common Emotions Expressed
One son objectively described his emotional experience in caring
for his mother in the late stage of dementia: "It's like being on a
emotional roller coaster, and in a 24-hour period, you experience
just about every emotion known to mankind." In their narratives on
caregiving, sons expressed five common emotions: love for their parent, pain and anguish, anger and resentment, sadness mingled with
compassion, and guilt. They also verbalized their caregiver stress and
burden. Many of the sons had difficulty putting their feelings into
words; some, though, were able to express their feelings articulately,
as demonstrated below.

Love for their parent was a common theme among many of the
sons. One 62-year-old son, who had retired early to care for his
mother, simply said, "Husbands and wives come and go. You can
always get a new one, but you only have one mother." Another 60-
year-old son more eloquently expressed his love for his mother in
this way.

The last month [of her life] was really not too good for her. She had her
eyes closed and was not responding to very much, but I did get one re-
sponse out of her. I was telling her one night how much I loved her and
I appreciated everything she had done for me in my lifetime. I said, "But

more importantly than that, I guess the thing I know more than any-
thing in my life is that you loved me, and that means a lot to me." And
she opened her eyes and she tried to talk, you know, like confirming
what I was saying, and I said, "I know. I understand." And that was the
last gesture of recognition that she made.

Pain and anguish over their parent's condition, seeing the person
they once knew and depended upon disappearing before their eyes,
was another common theme. A 60-year-old son discussed his visits
to his father in the nursing home: "Walking into the nursing home
is no problem. It's when I walk away. You know . . . the deterioration is still tough for me to deal with." A 46-year-old son whose
father had just died expressed similar emotions:

I never wanted to see my father as what he'd become. He was strong
physically. He was the macho image. I will always remember him pic-
tured in a sleeveless shirt, tan looking, wearing his Navy hat in the
Philippines, being trim and being muscular, and glistening in the sun
and being tan; and all of those things that evoke macho. And at the end,
here was this guy in this fetal position who had lost all kinds of weight,
who looked like he had just been let out of Dachau, and who was crying
and pleading. And that killed me. It still does. It still does.

As one man astutely summed up his feelings, "Everyone feels their
pain in their own way."

Anger and resentment, on many different levels and for many
different reasons, were also present in the interviews. One 47-year-
old son, who had helped his family face the facts about his mother's
illness, asked the proverbial question, "WHY?" He angrily stated,
"Why, why her. This was a woman who worked all of her life, took
care of and raised a family, was a good wife, and she had retired
when she was 60 to enjoy life."

Anger with the service-delivery system and its inability to help
in times of crisis was the paramount frustration of another son helping care for a dying father:

The system exacerbates what a disease does to a family. You can't get . . .
from the best sources, you can't get good answers or specifics. Half the

information isn't valid. And nobody has answers to the stuff. It is just so difficult. The whole thing just beats the family up terribly.

Other sons expressed anger and resentment at their situation and at the lack of assistance from other siblings. One 45-year-old son spoke of his attempts to help his parents; his mother was in the very early stage of dementia.

I'm damned if I do and I'm damned if I don't. I'm the one here in town helping and I'm the one that's to blame for something, everything or nothing. Then I try to fill in some of the details [for his sister] and then she doesn't want to hear it [his sister lives out of town]. I said, "I'm sorry, you can't hide from it just because you are almost 400 miles away. I have it every day and I'm not gonna let you sit out there and tell me 'I'm glad you're there.'" I'm not glad I am here, not when it's like this.

Guilt was also a common emotion many of these sons felt. They felt guilty for many reasons: guilt that they had not done enough for their ill parents, guilt about some past behavior toward their parents, and guilt for what this experience was doing to their families, wives, and children.

One 46-year-old son helping his mother care for his father admitted his feelings of guilt, saying, "There was never enough time to do what I felt I should have done. I let my mother carry too much of it 'cause she was strong, and so in my case I went to the point of the path of least resistance."

"I hollered at her! I hollered at her! Because she'd forget," one son commented about his behavior toward his mother, with whom he was living. "You regret hollerin' at people and things, you know. If you could only forgive 'em for whatever went on while they're alive, because it's too late when they're gone," he confessed.

Feelings of guilt were also voiced by an only child, who had moved back to Cleveland from out West with his wife to provide hands-on care to his mother. She was suffering from multi-infarct dementia. His was guilt about the sacrifices he was asking his wife to make.

I just feel terrible about stealing those years from my wife, those precious years. This is not what we had planned for our mid-fifies. It wasn't the direction we were heading in, and I just hope that somewhere in the future we'll be able to make up for that in some way or somehow. That's really the thing I regret most.

Feelings of sadness and compassion for their parents' situations also often permeated the interviews with the sons. One example of this sadness and compassion for his parents' situation was expressed by a man who was caring for both parents who had Alzheimer's disease. He voiced these feelings:

The emotional sense of sadness . . . it is just so overwhelming, just a sadness that I can't describe. It was too sad to see these very competent, capable, accomplished people—they were very successful in what they did, and they did it together.

More than half the sons, unlike the husbands, used the terms "stress" and "burden" to describe their emotional experiences with caregiving. One 35-year-old African-American son voiced those sentiments. He had moved into his mother's house to try to help her. He stated, "I'm putting so much in here that I am losing myself, you know? I'm really losing myself. I'm so stressed out."

A 53-year-old son caring for a father in the early stage of dementia was willing to discuss the burden of caregiving and a man's inclination to try to do it himself. He stated:

I really do think that men tend to isolate themselves. We do believe this myth that we're supposed to be able to do everything all on our own. "I'm a rock. I can do everything, and if I do take on this burden, then I'm gonna do it all by myself. I'm gonna roll up my sleeves and do it." And we sort of grow up with this notion.

Sons were more willing than husbands to verbalize and acknowledge the caregiver stress and burden they were feeling.

In summary, sons experienced a wide range of emotions—from love to burden and everything in between—as they took on the caregiving role for an ill parent. They were emotionally invested and involved in this caring process.

Loss

Loss was also a common theme expressed by sons. For some men, it was the loss of a person they loved. For other sons, it was a loss of personal space and freedom; for others it meant lost job opportunities. Some experienced all of these things, and struggled to overcome a compounded sense of loss.

One son described what he felt was the most difficult thing for him to deal with in the process of his mother's Alzheimer's disease: "I miss the person she was; she was somebody you could confide in—you could be yourself."

For a 53-year-old son, caring for his father in his home, the struggle was with his loss of space, privacy, and independence. He reflected on his loss:

We went from being pretty much a family where everybody was sort of independent. You could come and go as you want, and you didn't have to worry about anybody else. So, you go from this total freedom and dump in some dependency and everybody has to adjust. It's frustrating. Sometimes I'll want to work at home, and it's hard to work at home because he wants attention. And that's a normal human need, and so I don't get mad. I just feel like I don't have my own personal space like I used to.

A number of sons spoke of lost job opportunities, feeling unable to leave town to further their careers. They were putting their careers on hold for a while, and were uncertain what the long-term ramifications of this would be.

Dealing with Siblings

During the interviews, the sons discussed the roles their siblings played in the caregiving process and the impact the illness of the parent had on their relationships. There were four types of roles siblings played in the caregiving process. First, there was the group of siblings who equally shared the responsibility of caring for the parent. As one son in this group said, "I wouldn't want to be the sole caregiver for my father and neither would my brother." Most often "sharing the care" involved two equally supportive brothers. The second pattern depicted the converse of the first one. For numerous reasons, the son took total charge of the situation and provided almost all the care, with siblings doing a minimal amount of work and visiting the parent only sporadically. The third pattern was where the son provided the emotional and hands-on care to the parent while the other siblings handled the financial and legal aspects. And in the final pattern, the son provided mainly the emotional care and support services, such as transportation and financial advice, while a sister provided more of the hands-on care. This last pattern is the one most identified in other studies (see Chapter 1).

Having a parent with dementia affected the sibling relationships. For some siblings, their parent's illness brought them closer together. They talked more over the phone and saw each other frequently, sometimes daily. One son remarked, "I am talking to my brother more than I ever did before." Other times, the tensions brought on by the parent's illness reawakened old sibling rivalries, often accompanied by a sibling's refusal to accept responsibility in the parent's care, pushing the siblings further apart.

One 67-year-old son moved into his mother's home to help her after a hospitalization; his brother provided no assistance to their ill mother. He related the situation to us:

Finally I got hold of him [called his brother] late one evening around 11:00 because I told him, "I need help." He said, "Yes, yes, I'll be there." Wednesday, Thursday, and Friday went by, and I would call him every evening. Saturday morning, I called him and I said to him, "What in God's name is wrong with you? I've been asking you to come and you told me you're gonna come."

Some siblings were able to put past relationships aside for the sake of the parent; others could not. Very few sibling relationships appeared unaffected by the experience of caring for an ill parent.

Work Flexibility
A key factor that allowed many of the sons in this study to participate actively in caring for their ill parent was the amount of control and flexibility they had over their work hours. Sons who were business executives, salesmen, artists, professors, and blue-collar workers with seniority, having some control over their work schedules, used

this flexibility to their advantage. The sons who did not have that built-in advantage experienced more caregiver stress.

A 46-year-old son, helping a mother care for a sick father, said this about his situation with an already hectic work schedule:

The burden of our lifestyles is already pretty bad on a good day. I mean you are running for an airplane at 6:30 in the morning; you've been in three different cities and two different time zones. And you do that three or four times a week and on weekends. It's not a great lifestyle on a good day, and then to have this overlay of emotion-laden tragedy that's playing out; that takes an additional burden, toll on your time and strength.

Another son heads a family-owned corporation. He spoke of the advantages his job flexibility gives him while attempting to deal with his father's medical problems:

I mean, I would have to take weeks off to resolve this. Where in my position I don't have to worry about that because I am covered, but I can see where this [control over your hours] would be a necessity because there's no way you can run a job and deal with this at times.

Over half of the sons in this study helping to care for a parent with dementia had some flexibility in choosing the hours they worked.

Reversing the Roles

Sons often expressed difficulty in accepting the fact that they now had to take on roles and tasks that their parents used to do for them when they were children. In particular, the issues of bathing and driving were the most difficult for them to handle. One 59-year-old son whose father is in a nursing home said, "To be honest with you, I've been doing things that I didn't think I'd ever do for him of a personal nature. Like trying to put his teeth in so he can eat, or worst of all giving him a bath; doing things for him I just never, never thought I would be doing."

Things become even more complicated when it is a son trying to provide personal care to his mother. One 71-year-old African-American son described his attempts to try to wash his 96-year-old mother. He would tell her:

"Now, Mom, we got to do something here." She would say, "No, don't touch me." "I can't let you sit around the house all day and not let you be as clean as you want." So, I would be determined and take her into the bathroom and say, "Well, Mom, I'm not looking. I got the towel and said we're gonna get a little clean." This and that, but we worked it out.

Driving, especially if the ill parent was a man, was a particularly difficult situation for many of the sons to handle. Driving symbolizes much more to people than a mode of transportation; it also represents freedom, independence, pleasure, and status. To take the car keys away, especially from a man of that generation who had usually been the primary driver in the family, was a traumatic event for both father and son. Often, it was these fathers who had taught their sons how to drive, and who had taken the car keys away from them as teenagers if they used poor judgment. Sons often went into elaborate stories, with 10- to 15-minute narratives describing their attempts to convince their fathers to give up the car keys and stop driving.

Coming to terms with the fact that their parents were now in a stage of their illness that required the sons to take over such meaningful duties for them was one of the most difficult parts of this caregiving process for these sons.

Coping Strategies

There were four major coping strategies that sons talked about in their efforts to handle the emotional and physical demands of caring for a parent with dementia. These strategies were using a problem-solving approach, immersing themselves in their work, confiding in their wives, and finding solace and support in their religious convictions. Many of these sons used a combination of these strategies to aid them in their caregiving.

Using a problem-solving approach helped the sons to focus on the immediate issues, gather information, and strategize ways to find acceptable solutions, although as one son admitted, "The biggest frustration is there are no clear-cut solutions or answers." The men wanted to be prepared. Many sons used a search and seek method, best described by a 50-year-old son sharing the care of his father with his older brother:

I think what we have tried to do is to get as much information as is available. Seek out and search and talk with as many people as you can. Get as much information as is available on the disease to learn about it. Learn about the course of events about what to expect. I think education is the primary key. We have done a lot of research. I think we know what to expect. Things don't always happen in the way we think they're going to happen, but at least I don't think there has to be what I call any major surprises.

For many of the sons, escaping by immersing themselves in their work was an effective coping technique. Surprisingly, some sons found that the caregiver responsibility increased their work productivity, for it was the one time they could block out all thoughts of the problems and really focus on one thing without feeling guilty. One son responded about his coping strategy:

Being able to get lost in the pressures of work. Work with nothing else to distract you; it's all-consuming and you have to pull yourself away from it. It's this great sucking tunnel, and if you like it, you don't pull that hard away from it. You can fill all your available time with work.

For the married sons, the wives played the vital role of confidant and sole source of emotional support (a few siblings also played this role). Most sons did not discuss their parents' situation with other friends and relied solely on their wives for this support. Their wives, for the most part, did not provide the hands-on care or run the errands for the parent. The sons in the study describe them as pillars of emotional support. A 50-year-old son voiced these sentiments well, speaking about his wife's role:

When I am emotionally spent, because of this [the situation with his father], I've got my wife to talk with. When I get all tensed up and I go, "Jeez, oh, man, I feel so bad about this," and then we talk. We kind of go through it.

The last common coping strategy that many of the sons relied upon was their strong religious beliefs, their belief in God. When asked what helps him to cope, one son answered, "My religion more than anything else. I think it reduces stress because anytime I'll just go over to the cathedral near my office and sit there for 15, 20 minutes and think about things." For an African-American son caring for his 96-year-old mother, his belief in God was also a source of support and guidance. He said, "So, when things were going bad, I say, 'Hey, it'll come and the Lord will guide me whichever way it goes.'"

Paying Back and the Positive Impact of Caregiving

As difficult as the caregiving process was for the sons in this study, some could step back from their experience and discuss the positive outcomes that came from this ordeal. Sons talked about three positive aspects: a chance to "pay back" their parents for their care of them, a sense of purpose and satisfaction from simply being able to provide care to their parents, and the opportunity to provide a role model for their own children.

"Paying back" were the exact words that reoccurred many times in the dialogues with sons. This caregiving was an opportunity, as demanding, troublesome, and emotionally wrenching as it was, that gave them a chance to return, at least on a small scale, what their parent had done for them over the years. If not for their parent's dementia, they may never have had that opportunity. One 60-year-old son, caring for an ill mother, shared these thoughts:

It's just that I was pleased that I was able in some small way to be able to pay her back. I think if she had died of a heart attack, I would have never had the chance to say to myself in some small way I repaid her for what she did. Not that she ever made me feel like I had to, but I had to.

Sons caring for parents both in the early and late stages of dementia talked about the sense of satisfaction and purpose they received from the caregiving process. One son caring for his mother with early dementia voiced these sentiments: "It feels really good knowing my mother trusts me. I feel good that I, out of the family, have the abilities to do it." Another son expressed satisfaction derived from the meaning caregiving provided him: "After being in this for awhile, you start thinking what is the purpose [in life], and maybe the purpose is giving instead of getting. And so you give in some small way to somebody else who's important to you. So, that's what I mean by feeling a sense of satisfaction."

Being a role model for their children was also uppermost in many sons' minds, as they "shouldered their responsibility." The sons did not agree on the role their children should play in helping an ill grandparent, but the importance of the example they were setting for the children was a meaningful part of their experiences. One 46-year-old son, whose father had recently died, verbalized his thoughts:

I'm conscious that everything I do is a role model as a parent. Some good, some bad. But, I think they saw me trying. I think they saw me picking up what I felt was my burden. I mean that in a positive and loving way. And I think they saw me loving my parents and playing that out on a work level and an emotional level. I think they understood.

So, even during this "descent into the abyss," as one son described the experience of watching his father descend into Alzheimer's disease, sons can also see some affirming value.

Conclusion

This chapter reveals another perspective on son caregivers than that which is usually reported (see Chapter 1) and in that process broadens our awareness of the complexity of the caregiving experience for sons. The sons in this study varied in the tasks they were performing for their parents, from personal care to patient advocacy. Some sons provided support to mothers, others to fathers; some had active help from other siblings and some were doing it on their own. All, however, were committed to care for their parents. Caregiving may have taken place in their own home, in their parent's home, or in a nursing home, but these sons were actively participating in their parents' care. As one son aptly said, "The most important thing is just to get involved."

This group of sons shared similar experiences caring for a parent with dementia, common threads that bind them together. Their sense of duty, willingness to accept the devastating diagnosis early in the course of the illness, and confidence in their ability to take charge helped them to develop a workable care plan. However, as one son said, "The trouble with this disease is there are no good solutions."

Flexible work hours for many of the sons aided them, as they worked the demands of caregiving into their schedules. Effective coping strategies of problem solving, escaping into their work, turning to their wives or girlfriends for emotional support, and connecting with their religious background helped many of these sons through difficult times and decisions.

A particularly difficult decision, in which many sons were involved, was the determination of when their parents should stop driving. Throughout this process, sons were struggling with the emotions of seeing their parents "disappear before their eyes." They felt love, anger, pain, resentment, burden, sadness, and multiple levels of loss.

But the majority of the sons also felt a sense of satisfaction from this caregiving experience. They were able to "be there for their parent," and to pay him or her back for all the care the parent had shown them. The men were also very cognizant of their position as a role model for their own children.

These 30 very different sons had in common the experience of caring for a parent with dementia. It was this shared experience that made the narratives of the 30 sons come together and speak in a common voice.

Chapter Six
Toward a Typology of Son Caregivers

The 30 sons interviewed shared many similar experiences, yet they adapted to their caregiving roles in many different ways. These orientations helped them cope with the difficulties of caring for a parent with dementia, and provided them with direction and a sense of mission as they carried out the tasks of caregiving. From the narratives the sons shared with us, four distinct patterns of caregiving emerged. These four types of son caregivers we named "the dutiful son," "going the extra mile," "the strategic planner," and "sharing the care."

The four types share many characteristics and many of the themes discussed in Chapter 5, but the sons' approach to caregiving in each group was different. They used distinctive words to describe caregiving, and their actions were distinguishly different. Twelve narratives of sons' experiences will be described below to illustrate the differences among these four groups of sons.

"The Dutiful Son"

The sons in "the dutiful son" type had in common their sense of duty toward their parents. This was the driving force that motivated them to become actively involved in their care. The sons either shouldered the total responsibility of getting care for the parent, or were the moving force that spurred siblings to work together and make the arrangements for their parent's care. Throughout the narratives, they repeatedly mentioned their responsibility for their parents.

There were two variations of the dutiful son type: the dutiful sons whose sense of duty was strongly mingled with deep emotions of love, compassion, and sometimes anger and resentment, and the dutiful sons who accepted and shouldered their responsibility matter-of-factly. The differences in the two variations were the overriding emotions that accompanied the first group's sense of duty. Most often the emotion was the son's intense feeling of love for his ill parent, and this added another dimension to his feeling of duty. These sons used words and actions that expressed these feelings. The second group of sons accepted their responsibility as inherent to the role of son with little question or discussion, and their words and actions reflected this view. As one son in this second group said, "Why do I do take on this responsibility? I just do it. That's it." Narratives from sons who illustrate the different versions of the dutiful son are introduced below. Mr. Brown and Mr. Stein represent the first group of sons.

Mr. Brown

Mr. Brown is a slender, unmarried 41-year-old African-American man; after living out of town for a number of years, he returned home to be near his aging parents. He is a man of strong, complex emotions and has a certain philosophical proclivity. While discussing his return to his hometown, he said, "Now at age 41, you realize what is important and what is not." He is a systems analyst and has recently changed jobs, which meant a substantial cut in pay, but it gave him more flexibility in his job hours. This allows him more time to be available for his mother's needs. As he says, "You can't put a price on family. I was making more money in '87 than I am making now, but I got more peace of mind. I can arrange my schedule accordingly."

His mother is in the middle stage of dementia. She still recognizes him and his sister, but is having great difficulty communicating. As Mr. Brown said, "She understands what you're saying, but she can't express herself." She needs assistance in all areas of personal care.

The interview with Mr. Brown took place downtown at an old house in which he is living. His aim is to renovate the whole house, and he is currently working on the living and dining rooms. Sprinkled throughout these two rooms is some of the antique furniture his mother had restored. They shared a love for antiques.

He spends much of his spare time across the street with his mother. He had arranged for his mother to live with one of his neighbors, who is paid to care for her. He often stays there with her in the suite he had set up for her. This was an arrangement that seemed to be working, as he had recently taken his mother (with the help of his sister, who is a nurse) out of a nursing home. His father did not want the responsibility of caring for his wife and had placed her there. Mr. Brown poignantly described the situation:

My mother was dying there. I couldn't look at her. She was just giving up. I looked at her real good and I could see it in her eyes. I knew I just had to get her out of there. I even joked about kidnapping her from there. I was sitting on my back porch, explaining my situation to a neighbor, and not knowing what to do and she said, "Well, I'll help you, because I'm not working now. I'll do what I can do." I was ready to quit my job and I hate to say it, but go on welfare if I needed to, to take care of her!

This [arrangement] is a lot better than a nursing home. My sister is actively involved, too, but by my being so much closer, if sometimes the caretakers don't show up, I can fill in at times. My sister helps a lot. I've been blessed with some good people in my life.

Mr. Brown has been able to arrange for some home health aides to help his mother a few days a week, and his neighbor is there to supervise the care and make sure everything is going smoothly.

In discussing his feelings for his mother, he used the word "nurturing" as a way of describing their relationship.

My mother nurtured me. A child is not accountable for the parent-child relationship. The parent is, because the parent is the eldest and is supposed to guide. So, if a child grows up and is not close to the parent, don't blame the child. My mother nurtured that. She made very big sacrifices for us and she is not going to be here forever. So, I don't want her to leave this earth and not do my best for her. She made me who I am.

He has very mixed feelings toward his father, who he feels has forsaken his wife of 41 years. His father comes once a month for a very brief visit to bring her social security check. Mr. Brown laments:

It is a very sad situation. It's really sad and it hurts. I've learned to let my anger go. I told my sister, "Rather than disrespect my father, I don't want to disrespect him, because what goes around, comes around. I just don't have any contact with him. We have to concentrate on mother and work with her and help her to be as comfortable as she can." That's where I direct my energy now, because this is where she is getting the best care and the best love. I love her very much.

The most difficult part of the caregiving process for him to deal with is to see and to accept the change he sees in his mother, who was a warm, loving, outgoing person.

My mother was very outgoing. She would just get up and go. She worked very hard. And as difficult as it has been for me, I have to accept it. I'm so far better than I was like, early. When Mama cried, I cried. Nobody wants to see their mother sad.

I couldn't work too well at work. My emotions were going back and forth. I would be there looking at the computer screen and my mind would wander off to my mother's situation. I would just sometimes have to leave, go to the bathroom, because I would break down. And even when I came back, I was sitting there in a daze, not really concentrating. But, I decided I got to do what I got to do for her. That's the main thing.

What has helped him through the most difficult times are his friends and neighbors, his sister, and his belief in God. Mr. Brown confided:

I realize even in a dark hour, there's still some light. It's just unbelievable some of the good people that have been put into our lives. My sister is a very strong girl. I think she got that from Mama. I mean there were times I would break down and she would say, "Now look, let's look at it this way." And I do believe in God. I definitely do. I pray and thank God every day. And my belief is, I'll do as much as I can, and after that point, God can just step in and do something.

His advice for other son caregivers is:

Things aren't always as bad as they feel. The main thing is we all have our own way of accepting it, but the sooner you accept it, the better you

can deal with the care of the individual. You've got to come to that
realization. And realize you are not God. You are going to need other
people. You are going to need the advice of the Alzheimer's Association
and all the reading material they have. Get the power of attorney and
get all that stuff in place. We're human and we can only do so much.

Mr. Brown's narrative illustrates his strong sense of duty and
devotion toward his mother, as well as a wide range of other com-
peting feelings. Certainly not all the sons in this group went as far as
taking their mother out of a nursing home, but the depth of their
emotions and their sense of duty were the focal parts of their narratives. Mr. Stein, whose narrative is presented below, also felt that
strong sense of duty to care for his mother, blended together with
his deep sense of love for her.

Mr. Stein

Mr. Stein, 43 years old, is a jogger whose physical activity is a method
of coping with the mounting stress in his life. He is an accomplished
musician whose busy life included teaching, performing, and a fledg-
ling record company. Now, he has taken on much of the responsibility for overseeing his mother's care. He is white and the middle child,
with a 46-year-old sister and a 33-year-old brother, both of whom
also live in town. His mother is 81 years old and entering the middle
stage of dementia. His father is still alive, but according to Mr. Stein,
"My parents never had a good marriage. My mother should have
left 40 years ago. My father is selfish and immature and can't be
trusted to care for my mother. He is ill equipped to care for my
mother as her condition worsens."

Yet to Mr. Stein's surprise, his father is trying to care for her. He
helps her get washed and fed, but when things get too difficult, he
will just walk out and leave her by herself. One night he left and
went to a hotel without telling anyone. Mrs. Stein had no idea what
had happened to her husband, but she was able to call her son for
help.

Mr. Stein cannot rely much on his siblings for help either; both of them are in denial and cannot handle their mother's
situation. His brother is immobilized by the experience. Mr. Stein
said:

My brother just zones out. He can't—He can't do anything. My father describes him when he comes for a visit . . . he lays on the floor, eats something, and watches television for a half an hour, and leaves. I think he would like to help, and he actually went with me down to the Social Services. I told him, "I really need you to do this so I don't end up resenting you." I mean, I was clear about what I wanted from my brother. I wanted my brother to have a little responsibility, but it didn't happen. I didn't expect anything from my sister, because I knew it wouldn't happen. She just gets hysterical. I think human beings do two things when they're coping with things. They either blank out or they accept it.

So it's Mr. Stein who has taken time off from work to arrange for services for his mother, Meals on Wheels and adult day care services three times a week. His parents' income makes them eligible for some countywide in-home services. If decisions are to be made or action to be taken, Mr. Stein is the one to do it.

He has arranged for the financial control of her bank accounts, to the relief of his father, because she would not sign anything for her husband. As Mr. Stein states matter-of-factly:

I'm the only person she trusts at this point in the family. So, I've accepted that. But it also feels good knowing my mother trusts me, whether it's something that relates from the illness now or prior, there's still that acknowledgment. And I do feel good that I, out of the family, have the abilities to do it.

In talking about his motivation for caring for his mother, it became clear that accepting this responsibility comes from his deep love for her, not because no one else was able to handle it. It was not by default that he stepped into this role. Mr. Stein and his mother had a very warm and loving relationship, and he always felt supported by her.

I love my mother and I always have, and she was very supportive of me. As a young child I was a little bit different. Didn't do well in school, but did have this ability in music. My father didn't support it at all—wanted me to go into business and whatever. But we [his mother and himself] were always pretty close, though we're not a close family. My caregiving is based on love, though I freely admit there's times it's the last thing I want to do, just to go over there. My wife wishes she could do something, but she just gets so depressed when she visits and my father isn't nice, so I generally go over by myself and spend a couple of hours. Sometimes it's like insanity on a daily basis. But if my brother and sister were helping out, I still would be doing this. There was no question in my mind that I was going to do this.

Continuing talking about his mother, Mr. Stein said:

I still remember my mother, not this—I mean, I look at this person, and the physical changes are so dramatic and every now and then . . . Last week, we sat out on the front stoop because she wanted to talk about something, and I remember being that little kid laying in her lap looking at her. There was that connection there. It was brief. It's funny how you just sort of remember little tidbits. She always was a very calming force in my life.

One day she started to say to me something about getting old and stuff, and I just said to her, "It's okay, Ma. It's part of the process. It's part of the learning experience." She just smiled, and sometimes there are those connections.

Mr. Stein estimates he spends roughly 10 to 12 hours a week at his parents' home. He works about 60 hours a week, so it's difficult to go over more often, yet he talks to his mother multiple times a day, although often she can't remember speaking to him. And he always comes when he can. He has no children, so he does have more control over his time. He finds his mother remarkably understanding. He said, "I think she feels much better knowing that someone's really trying to get there for her."

Alzheimer's disease has had an impact on Mr. Stein's life. He is very stressed:

Any phone call that comes very late or very early, I jump out of bed and expect the worst. I've truly been affected by the fact that anything can happen at any time. I have to be prepared somehow. But I won't let it interfere to the point of anything in my work. So I carry a lot of tension with me.

He has multiple ways of coping that seem to relieve some of the stress. Exercise is a big help to him. "I always feel better afterwards. I feel much more on a neutral level. If something comes along, I'm gonna handle." His wife is also a big support. He stated, "I have a very supportive wife. For example, if I need to go off at 7:30 in the morning to do something for my mother, my wife understands. So, that's been very helpful."

Work, too, offers him an escape. He can get lost in his music. He shared with us, "If I can get into practicing, you know, I go off into another world. And once I get into my teaching, except for an emergency, I don't let anything interfere." He knows he is lucky to have flexibility in his job:

I am very fortunate that I am my own boss. Even if I am teaching one day and one of these calamities come up, I can call my students and tell them there's been a family emergency. They understand, and I'll make up the lesson some other time. I have the flexibility that most men do not have.

Friends are also a source of support for him. He has a friend who has also been caring for a parent with Alzheimer's disease. She has little sibling help, and works full-time. They share stories and helpful suggestions with each other, and have often joked, "It's too bad we aren't in the same family." Respite, or time away, has also been very helpful in relieving the stress and burdens of caregiving for Mr. Stein. Just getting away for a weekend with his wife recently made a world of difference for him. His mother understood; he left a note to remind her.

The hardest part of the experience with dementia for Mr. Stein is that his mother, "who was such a sweet and kind person," now seems to be suffering. "She's so miserable and cries all the time; she has taken this tormented direction. There is nothing pleasant in life for her anymore."

When asked to give advice for other caregivers, Mr. Stein's first suggestion was to get involved with the Alzheimer's Association or another social service agency familiar with the services available to individuals with dementia. He remarked:

Get involved with a social worker or the Alzheimer's Association to get some solid information and find out what services are available. Find out the financial situation of the parents, because that's where the reality is. I think a lot of us kids just don't know how much money their folks had. I had no idea. I think that's probably the most helpful thing. And simply be patient. Acknowledge that you are going to feel rotten. You are going to. Being told about what is going to happen, point-blank, right up front is probably the best. Just get that information right up front. And it is different for everybody. I would like to have been told, "This is going to be tough." But the doctors are so afraid to say the word "Alzheimer's."

Mr. Stein ended the interview by stating that merely sharing your experiences with others can be helpful to you. And seeking professional help should not be ruled out.

You may need some professional advice and need to go and talk to someone. Nobody talks about that, particularly if you are stuck in that situation. And I think people my age are more open in general to doing that sort of thing.

Mr. Stein and Mr. Brown illustrate the type of dutiful son who takes on the caregiving duties for a parent. Both men accepted their responsibilities, and would have done it with or without the assistance of siblings. Yet, strongly mingled with this sense of duty was the deep emotion of love for their ill parents. The strength of this affection was the tie that bound these sons to the caregiving role for their parents.

The second variation of "the dutiful son" is illustrated by the two narratives below. These sons also accept the duty and responsibility of caring for an ill parent, but with the themes of loyalty and filial obligation overshadowing emotional love. They approach caregiving "matter-of-factly," and distinguish themselves from the previous narratives.

Mr. McLaughlin

Mr. McLaughlin is a white 55-year-old artist who has lived in many of the art centers of the world. For years, he had been a financially successful businessman. As he entered his forties, he decided it was time to follow his artistic inclinations; otherwise he might never. He has a confident and assured manner, and makes decisions with much ease. He was the fourth son from a family of eight children, most of whom remained in town.

His mother had been diagnosed with Alzheimer's disease 11 years ago, and she was in the end stage of the disease. His parents had moved into a small mother-in-law's suite attached to the home of one of his sisters. However, after his father died, it became too much for his sister to care for their mother and her own eight children. Mr. McLaughlin felt a strong responsibility toward his mother and the need to help out his sister.

On one of his visits home, it became apparent to him that his mother was gradually getting worse, more confused and forgetful. He called a family meeting to discuss the situation.

The reaction of the other locals [children] was, "It's not our problem." They weren't even helping out my sister on weekends. As they did not want any responsibility and I was used to getting things done and could paint anywhere, I said, "Fine." That's when I became captain. I told my other siblings [other than his sister], "I don't want to hear anything about her [their mother's] finances, where she is, her care, whatever. I mean, if you want to do it, fine, but if I'm in charge, I'm in charge." We set up a trust to take care of my mother's care and I am the sole trustee. On the advice of the physician, we started discussing nursing homes; we formed a little task force and looked at 15 nursing homes in the area.

When his mother moved into a nursing home, Mr. McLaughlin knew he would have to move back to his hometown. He looked for space to open a studio and moved into the mother-in-law's suite. He was not married and had an occupation that allowed much flexibility of location and working hours. He reflected back on the move home:

I knew I would have to be there. I mean physically in the area, to kind of watch over her care, to visit every day at the nursing home, go and feed a meal, and do volunteer work there. My attitude was that if I was in charge, I had to be around physically. I am the one constant factor in her life over her years in the nursing home. My mother may not know who I am, but I am a familiar face.

Mr. McLaughlin goes every day to visit his mother and feed her the evening meal. He speaks with the nursing home staff and checks on her care, and he has "adopted" other residents whom he visits daily.

Mr. McLaughlin has accepted matter-of-factly the responsibility for his mother. He didn't think it was fair that his sister was saddled with the care of his mother, and he felt a need to pay back his mother for her care of him.

I didn't want her to feel she [his sister] was stuck with it. So it was kind of to ease that burden. She had mother so long at home and went through this with very little support from the rest of the family. I have now been able to psychologically take that burden off of her, 'cause it is a burden, and make her feel like it's okay. She didn't give up. I just came in and took over. I also feel like I am giving something back, which is a good feeling. I do feel like I am paying my dues.

Mr. McLaughlin also wonders what the experience must be like for his mother, if she is aware at times of her situation, and this has kept him returning daily to the nursing home. His compassion for her situation is evident from the following dialogue.

It would be much easier on me if I thought she was in outer space, if she were totally not with us, but the idea that even occasionally she has lucid moments and knows what her problems are and where she is and who we are makes me crazy. A consciousness that is locked in there, that's even aware part of the time, what a terrifying thing that must be. So, it's made me operate on the basis that there is an aware consciousness at least part of the time. I go every day because of the fear that there's a person trapped in there who needs to be comforted.

So duty, acceptance, and responsibility are major themes that recur in Mr. McLaughlin's narrative, as well as other "dutiful sons" who fall into this group. They take on the responsibilities and accept what comes with it. As Mr. McLaughlin commented:

I don't have to do this. And when it really gets to me, I take off for awhile. I mean it upsets me that she has this disease. I know what the disease does. I mean, I have done my homework. But it's like, okay, you've just got to deal with it. Life is full of experiences to which you must rise to the occasion.

Mr. McLaughlin has advice for other sons who are starting to get involved in the care of a parent with dementia:

Get a living will and durable power of attorney signed, sealed, and delivered as fast as possible. Go look at nursing homes because the question is not gonna be "whether," it's gonna be "when." I would look at earlier placement rather than later, when they're more adaptable to the change of moving into a group environment and can enjoy the stimulation of the programs. So, I would say, do your homework and find out about the Alzheimer's stuff. It's very complicated. And keep smiling.

Another example of this "dutiful son" type is Mr. Lombardo. Like Mr. McLaughlin and Mr. Brown, he had a strong sense of duty and responsibility to care for his parent. But like Mr. McLaughlin, his motivation stems from a sense of duty that each child owes a parent.

Mr. Lombardo

Mr. Lombardo is a white, married 60-year-old retired schoolteacher with a wonderful sense of humor. He often used this humor during the interview to describe some of the difficult, at times funny, situations he had with his father. His father is now 85 years old and in the middle stage of dementia.

Mr. Lombardo is an only child, and to best understand his situation, he spent some time discussing his early relationship with his father. Mr. Lombardo stated that he always had a "rocky relationship" with his father, who was quite domineering. Mr. Lombardo's mother died when he was a teenager, and it was difficult for his father to raise him alone. He grew up in a small rural town, where his father was the high school football coach. Mr. Lombardo said of his father:

He was a football coach, and that was practically his whole life. He didn't understand raising teenagers or providing a warm supportive family environment. Unfortunately, I went to the school where he coached and had to play football. If we ever lost a game, of course, it was my fault. There was always friction between us and fortunately for me at that time, he had brothers and sisters, and his parents were alive. And I lived with his parents for a short period of time.

When Mr. Lombardo graduated from high school, he went away to college, but not the college his father expected him to go to, and he never returned home. He married soon after finishing college, started teaching in a school district in a different part of the state, and saw his father five or six times a year. Despite their differences, Mr. Lombardo always felt a deep sense of responsibility and loyalty to his father. There was never a doubt that he would assist his father if he ever needed any help.

To get a better understanding of his father's condition, Mr. Lombardo kept a written record of his father's increasing difficulties, as well as his own reactions to them. Mr. Lombardo said, "I'm the type of person who likes to know what I'm dealing with. I felt in order for me to know what to do, I ought to know what I'm dealing with first. But right now, truthfully, it's become a form of therapy."

Mr. Lombardo began to realize something was wrong when his father kept phoning long distance to ask him to handle more and more of his financial matters. This was completely out of character for him. His father was "fiercely independent" and handled all of his own financial matters. But now his father was misplacing money and safety deposit box keys, and didn't remember banking transactions. Then he put kerosene in his car instead of gas and completely ruined the engine. The situation was becoming progressively worse, yet when his father came for brief visits, he was still able to hide the forgetfulness and confusion, for the most part.

Finally, Mr. Lombardo realized something was really wrong. His father's behavior, Mr. Lombardo said, "had always been a little odd. He lived alone, never had a phone, and was never much interested in any material possessions. He always wanted to be ready to pack up and go in 15 minutes and take all his possessions with him." Yet Mr. Lombardo felt his father's behavior was becoming progressively more bizarre. Mr. Lombardo decided to travel to his hometown and see for himself what was happening. At this time he discovered that

his father had been cashing his Social Security checks and not remembering that he had done so. He would practically give away all
his money to strangers on the street, who he said were his best friends.
He wasn't eating properly, his hygiene was very poor, and he was
getting into arguments with everyone. With his wife's help, Mr.
Lombardo packed up his father's belongings and brought him to his
house and then tried to get him medically evaluated. His father hated
doctors and saw no use for them. This led to a poignant but humorous description of how Mr. Lombardo arranged to take his father
for a geriatric assessment.

*There is only one person in this whole world that my father looks up to,
that's his older brother, Roy. My Uncle Roy is now 94 years old and was
my father's football coach in college. So, I called him and explained
what was going on. He wouldn't believe me at first, saying, "Oh, your
dad's just getting old." But after describing all his bizarre behavior, he
agreed to help. I had to prearrange everything. We told my father he was
meeting Roy for lunch. Roy was waiting at the entrance of the medical
center to greet us. My son—because he won't do anything I ask him to do
and is always mad at me—hops out of the car and says, "Come on
Grandpa, let's go. There's Uncle Roy." My son and daughter escorted him
into the building before he could read any of the signs. My father starts
to look around the medical clinic and turns to his brother and says,
"God, Roy, you sure pick strange restaurants. What the hell kind of restaurant is this?" Finally we got him in there and got the assessment.
Once he figured out where he was, he was terrible. His brother and I
had to sit there through all the tests with him. He made such a fuss that
finally his 94-year-old brother said to him, "Goddamn it Joe, what did
I use to tell you. Remember when we were playing [football] against the
WB team and I knew the play was coming towards you and I'd make
the signal and you'd make the tackle every time? Well, I'm doing that
now. I'm making that signal. Do what the doctor says." Then my father
would do what the doctor asked.*

At the family meeting with the medical team, Mr. Lombardo
was told his father had "probable Alzheimer's." He immediately
bought six books on the topic, and the whole family started reading
and trading them around. Mr. Lombardo said:

We started reading up on it just to find out exactly what we were dealing with, and then I, of course, was kind of in denial too. Just for a long time I couldn't talk about it without tears. Here's this guy, who was fiercely independent, never smoked or drank and now he didn't even know where he was.

At the conference with the social worker and doctor, I told them I was gonna try to keep him home with me. Knowing our relationship, they didn't think it was going to work, but I had to try. It lasted five weeks because he was going to hit me on several occasions.

After that, Mr. Lombardo tried several arrangements, but his father kept saying, "I want to go home." They tried an assisted-living facility, and Mr. Lombardo agreed to pay extra for an aide to come in and help bathe his father; his father would not let Mr. Lombardo himself help. He furnished the rooms with things he thought his father would like, but this living arrangement did not work out either. During this time Mr. Lombardo felt quite guilty. He stated:

I felt like such a rat. I'm doing all these things that he didn't want me to do. All he kept saying was "I want to go home." The assisted living lasted eight months, and only because I was there half the time. It's a wonder they didn't charge me rent. But in those eight months, I learned to accept.

What helped Mr. Lombardo cope was learning more about the disease. He attended some educational workshops on Alzheimer's disease, read profusely on the subject, and attended a few sessions of a support group. His wife was supportive of his efforts, but she was dealing with the ill health of her own parents. He also found it particularly helpful to hold family meetings a couple times a year. He had started this before his father's illness, to discuss other family issues, but these meetings became a central part of planning for his father's care. Mr. Lombardo's wife and their three children and their spouses all attended these family meetings. It's from such a meeting that his son offered to care for his grandfather. He had always been the favorite grandchild, and he and his grandfather had a special relationship. The grandson's wife is in the health care field and has experience caring for elderly people. So the family agreed on financial arrangements that would pay for the care, and loaned the grandson money to buy a house that would provide a suitable environment for the grandfather. "At least," Mr. Lombardo said, "you can't say that we didn't try."

The motivating factor for Mr. Lombardo throughout this difficult ordeal with his father was his sense of responsibility:

I have a responsibility to my father, and I think we all have responsibilities to one another. I guess I am being as responsible as I can be in a bad situation. To tell you the truth, the thought did cross my mind to just take this guy back to his home and dump him off; he gave us such a bad time. But, I couldn't do that. And I think another thing too is I am setting an example for my kids. My kids have told me, "Dad, you are doing a great job."

Mr. Lombardo's final thoughts in the interview offered advice to other caregivers:

I think my first word of advice would be without a doubt to get a handle on the financial situation. You have to know what you are dealing with. Then you need to get [a medical] evaluation and get professional help. And you'd better get an attorney, because the laws are getting more and more complicated. I would say you have to get organized and accept the situation. And don't forget that sense of humor.

These four sons, Mr. Brown and Mr. Stein, and Mr. McLaughlin and Mr. Lombardo, represent the two groups of sons that comprise the category of "the dutiful son." They all have illustrated, through their words and actions, that they have taken on the role of caregiver to a parent. They have hired help or had friends and family assist, but they have shouldered the main responsibility and made the final decisions for the care. It was this sense of duty that motivated them and guided their actions. Mr. Brown's and Mr. Stein's motivation was a deep love and emotional commitment to their parents. Mr. McLaughlin's and Mr. Lombardo's motivation was a strong sense of family commitment, and acceptance that this was a role they needed to take. All four sons have been able to integrate that care into their present lifestyle.

"Going the Extra Mile"

The sons that typify the "going the extra mile" group went a step beyond the roles and actions of the "dutiful son" group. The "going the extra mile" type have brought their parents into their households, or moved back to town into their parents' homes to deliver hands-on personal care. They have made multiple sacrifices in their lives to care for their parent, and have put their own personal lives on hold. In essence, they took on the role of a "spouse caregiver." They speak of devotion to their parents, as well as an overwhelming sense of duty, and guilt if they had not taken on this role. Like the husband caregivers, however, they mention feelings of social isolation; unlike the husbands, they acknowledge caregiver stress and burden. They have little outside help, and the care is handled mainly by themselves or in conjunction with other siblings. Only as a very last resort, when they can go no further in the care, will they consider a nursing home. Interestingly, this group of six sons all had Catholic upbringings, and some were still quite religious. The three narratives presented below illustrate some of the unique characteristics of this type of son caregiver and how they adapted to their caregiving role.

Mr. Florenzo

Mr. Florenzo is an energetic, compassionate, white, 42-year-old man, the youngest of two brothers. Fourteen years ago, he moved his parents into town to live with him, and the parents intended to spend their winters in Florida. His parents were getting older, and he felt he should be available to provide them with the support they might need. His older brother, who was living in the same town as his parents, was not able to provide their parents with that help. Mr. Florenzo is now the director of a large, nonprofit agency and has recently married.

"Everything was going according to plan," and then eight years ago his mother was diagnosed with Alzheimer's disease. Mr. Florenzo spoke fervently about his experiences caring for an ill parent, and the difficulties he encountered as a son trying to be the sole provider. He had to learn new roles, and often had to deal with the disbelief of many health care providers that he (a son) could be a serious, competent caregiver. His father has since also developed dementia.

Reflecting on his mother's diagnosis he said:

The dynamic of the three of us living together began to truly change. There was a role reversal, and they were becoming increasingly dependent upon me. And we had a wonderful relationship, but you know just subtly you notice that there was a shift in dependency. My mother and I were very close; we were very close and I began compensating for her. It was an unspoken kind of thing. I did the cooking, laundry, all of the things my mother was a star at—managing the house, and keeping the ship in a state of float, so to speak.

Mr. Florenzo began taking on the roles of a spousal caregiver. His parents were a very traditional Italian couple, and as he said, "My father was clueless about how to do all this, but the expectation was still there on his part that everything would always be done the way they were. He was still working part-time and didn't want to deal with it." As time passed, Mr. Florenzo found himself taking on more and more of those roles, even cooking the traditional Sunday spaghetti dinner.

I'd cook when I got home from work. We sat around the dinner table and pretended everything was the same. Saturday and Sundays were totally consumed with what you had to do. It got to a point where I was bathing her, I was feeding her, I was cutting up her food. Everything was hyper-routinized. If anything deviated, it just threw the whole balance off, so my whole goal in life was to keep one day blended into the next. I didn't sleep more than five hours because you are afraid of what you're going to find when you get up and get out. And the thought of home health care just wasn't even in the picture at that point because first of all, there was some denial on my part that I didn't need it. I thought oh, I can do this. Sure, I can do this.

Like many of the husband caregivers, Mr. Florenzo was trying to do it all on his own. He was deeply committed to caring for his mother. When asked what helped to get him through this period, he said:

You just did what you had to do. I lived from day to day, and I didn't think about long range, or what it's going to be like in six months. I wasn't walking away from it. I couldn't. It was that deep commitment or whatever it is. It was just so deeply grounded in me that I wouldn't.

He had much resentment toward his brother, who would call and offer to help, but would never follow through. Mr. Florenzo voiced his resentment, anger, and frustration in the following way:

He [his brother] just didn't want to have anything to do with it. We would have big fights on the phone. He would say, "Well, what can I do?" And I would get furious with him. I remember distinctly one night I said, "Unless you're willing to come here and figure out how we're gonna get mom to brush her teeth and how you're gonna con her into putting a clean pair of clothes on, then we don't have anything to talk about. Now, if you want to help do that, because that's how you can help me." Well, he didn't want to do that. I had no relief.

He continued explaining the situation:

So, okay we have a deteriorating mother, a matriarch, as strong as anything. We've got a father who is emotionally just not dealing with it well at all, in lots and lots of denial. And you got another son who just wasn't around. And I felt like I was in the middle trying to hold it together, but this once emotionally close family was coming apart.

Eventually he admitted and accepted that he couldn't handle it alone and needed help. At first, they used a home health aide, but eventually he had to move his mother into a nursing home. The sense of guilt and failure that surrounded this decision still troubles him:

My mother was getting worse, progressing into the disease. She absolutely could not be left alone, and had to be lifted into the bathtub. The home health aide was coming at seven in the morning and would work until four. Then my Dad would come home from wherever he went and he would have the responsibility from four until six. Then I'd get home. We'd finish dinner and go through the drill of the pajamas, go to the bathroom, and all that stuff, but it was getting worse. We couldn't care for my mother anymore at home. And I didn't want to face this, and my dad definitely didn't want to face this. I really had to look at nursing homes, and finally I did. I had failed at being a caregiver, because if I had succeeded, we wouldn't be where we are. Now, I know that isn't true, but there's a piece of me that felt that. So there is a lot of guilt associated with it.

Mr. Florenzo also talked about his sense of social isolation and sacrifices. He could not maintain friendships; people his own age did not understand the situation. He did not have time to put into relationships, especially romantic ones. His professional life was also affected.

My ability to have relationships was very limited. I had lots of professional relationships because of the nature of the work I do, but in my personal life, I had a very, very small circle of friends. People don't understand it. My peers don't understand it because most of them have not gone through this. I had no one to talk to. I didn't feel a support system. Romantic relationships didn't last. I hurt myself personally and I hurt myself professionally. I think it limited my options. My options were shut down. In a lot of ways, I sacrificed a lot.

Yet, throughout this narrative, Mr. Florenzo never lost the compassion he felt for his mother, and then for his father, who developed similar symptoms. He also referred often to the sense of satisfaction and enrichment he received from this experience. He viewed it as a growth experience for him, "A blessing in disguise which I would do all over again."

The emotional sense of sadness was overwhelming. It was too sad to see these very competent, capable, accomplished people. Really, my mother and father were very successful. We were very close. My mother was a well-educated woman, and she was very smart. We shared a lot together intellectually. We read a lot. Well, we couldn't share those things anymore. It was so sad when I think about that. Yet I was strengthened by the experience. Emotionally, I don't think I would be as strong as I am today if it weren't for that. I think it is the most enriching thing that has happened to me. It's a special kind of blessing. I think very few are chosen in this world to experience some things like this. And I feel, as awful

as it was—and it was—I gained a much deeper understanding about
life and about love.

Mr. Florenzo's parents are now both in a nursing home, and
he visits them daily. His narrative illustrates the unique characteristics of this group of son caregivers. These are the sons who have
"gone the extra mile," who some would say went "beyond the call
of duty," though these sons would disagree with that statement.
They were very similar to the husband caregivers in their roles and
lives. They provided regular, personal care to their ill relatives, sacrificed much in their personal and professional lives, and experienced feelings of social isolation; however, unlike the husband
caregivers, they voiced their caregiver burden and stress. Their parents' care was their priority.

Mr. Florenzo concluded his narrative with advice for health care
professionals. He encourages health care professionals to become
aware that there are sons who are competent, concerned, and capable of providing hands-on care to ill parents. He complained that
he was not taken seriously.

It was just like they [particularly women professionals] were humoring
me. I don't know how else to characterize it, but they questioned that
you would even be in the least bit involved or concerned or interested in
all of this. What would I know from caring, bathing? I resent being
treated like a [19]60's kind of guy. And I'm talking about hip-with-it-
now kind of women and professionals in this field.

Many health care professionals did not expect Mr. Florenzo to be so
committed to caring for parents.

The next narrative also illustrates the "going the extra mile" type
of son. The characteristics are the same, though the situation is different. The next son is providing care, with assistance from siblings,
for his mother.

Mr. Polanski

Mr. Polanski is a tall, slender, white 32-year-old stockbroker. His mother
was diagnosed with early onset Alzheimer's disease 11 years ago, when
Mr. Polanski was just finishing college and still living at home. He is

one of seven siblings in a devout Catholic family. His father still works full-time, but takes minimal responsibility for his wife's care. According to Mr. Polanski, his father does not have the personality or patience to give their mother the care the children want her to have. As Mr. Polanski says, "He loves her, and Mom likes to hear his voice, but we've [the children] never felt comfortable just having him there by himself." The six children (one daughter is not involved) provide the hands-on care to their mother. Mr. Polanski stated:

I come from a big family and we never really considered a nursing home or anything like that. We went through all the stages of taking care of my mom just down the line of progression. Everyone kind of pitches in here or there. We've never really had any sort of outside help; it's all been family members taking care of her. We do just about everything for her. We love our mom and want the best for her.

While describing how the care is divided among the siblings, he stated, "It just sort of evolved over the years." Mr. Polanski (one of two brothers in the family) is the decision maker, breadwinner, and "relief pitcher" for the caregivers on the weekends. He works full-time, yet his job provides him with some flexibility in his hours as long as he "produces and meets his sales goals." He maintains two houses and an apartment, where he now lives. He moved his mother and father into his house as his mother's condition worsened because his house and neighborhood were quieter for her. He continued to live there for awhile, but decided it would be best if he moved to an apartment. He really had to focus on his work because it was very expensive taking care of her. He said, "I'd like to spend more time with my mom, but if I don't work to make money, we're not going to be able to keep taking care of her."

His two unmarried sisters, both in their late twenties, provide the hands-on care to their mother during the week, and he and his married siblings take shifts caring for their mother on the weekends. He takes the 9-to-5 shift on Saturdays and Sundays. Mr. Polanski provides his sisters with a house to get away from their caregiving duties on the weekends. Mr. Polanski and his siblings are committed to caring for their mother this way, and their devotion and respect for her motivates them. As Mr. Polanski said:

She was just a really great person. Never, ever raised her voice with any-body. Just a really excellent, excellent mother—really the greatest person I ever met. Honest to God, I'm not just saying that because she is my mother. She was always a great listener, a great friend. Just real strong emotionally, mentally, always knew the right thing to say; a good, religious person.

But guilt is also a motivating factor for Mr. Polanski. Caring for his mother is something that he wants to do, but also something he feels he must do. Reflecting on this feeling he said, "Guilt, yeah—a lot of guilt. I feel it's better for me to just suck it up and work harder or get stronger than to carry around guilt. Guilt is very fatiguing for me."

This dedication comes with much sacrifice, and Mr. Polanski is very cognizant of his sisters' and his own sacrifices.

It comes almost to a point where we are burned out, but there is no time to be burned out. I have not had time for myself and I am 32 years old. I haven't lived for the last 10 years. You sacrifice a lot of your own life, really. I'd work to five, go to my mom's right after work in my suit at 6:00 and help feed her dinner till 8:30. But I am going to get even with life; when my mom is gone, I'll take a year off, and I figure that will catch me up. I wouldn't plan anything. I'd just go.

My youngest sister is 27 and she has been always taking care of mom since the age of 16. She was the youngest and most available. She never had a full-time job. She's always been there. She went to college through all this, but didn't have the luxury of going away for four years. My other sister gave up her job to take care of Mom.

Social isolation also is a result of this commitment to caring for his ill mother, as Mr. Polanski states:

Most people my age now all have families. At first everyone wanted to go out. I never could. I'd say, "I'll meet you at 10:30 when I'm done," if I wasn't sleeping over at my mom's. It definitely affects your social life. You feel a bit lonely because even if you try to have a girlfriend, they never really understand. It hurts that nobody . . . and you try to deal with this mentally that "I can conquer it by myself," because you can't let yourself feel hurt. You just get through it, and you get through it, and you get through it. Socially, it is tough because I've missed a lot, I think.

A number of different strategies help Mr. Polanski cope with his caregiving responsibilities. First of all, learning to take his caregiving experience a day at a time or a month at a time has been enormously helpful to him. Mr. Polanski has learned that you have to "just go with the flow and whatever comes will come." It amazes him that 10 years have gone by and he is still able to provide the care.

Time away also helps. He occasionally takes a few days away, though when he does he feels he is letting his sisters down. "You feel boy, I'm having this few days' vacation, but my sisters have to pick up the slack for me because I couldn't handle it." An occasional game of golf gives him some respite, as does an evening out at a sports bar.

Just having a beer and mindlessly watching a game I find comforting. I also look forward to Friday and Saturday nights to go out and not to have to make any plans; just to go out. Just to have free time if I want to work out or if I want to spend time with my nephew or just do nothing.

His religion has also been a support for him. Mr. Polanski shared his thoughts with us: "I'm a Christian, a Catholic. I don't follow all the rules and regulations, but I do believe in being Christ-like—though I don't do a perfect job of it. But, I do believe in doing the right thing and a good example is you try to ask, what would Christ do?"

Perhaps what helps him most through the stresses of caregiving, however, is his sense of accomplishment and satisfaction.

My mom would be incredibly proud of me. She really would. I mean, I get satisfaction—sometimes people say or the doctor at the clinic says, "You guys are doing a great job. You're really a great family." When people who kind of know how long my mom's been sick or how long's we've been taking care of her say, "You're really a good person. You really sacrifice a lot." It makes me feel good. I've done that for my mom. It's a great feeling. There's definitely satisfaction involved.

For any sons who are starting to become involved in the care of a parent with dementia, Mr. Polanski offers this advice:

I think I'm lucky because I love my mother so much. But if there was another son who really loved his mother and wanted to take care of her and wanted to make her feel good, I would just say, "God's challenging you now and get your priorities in place. You can always do other things later. Try to do the right thing and if you feel taking care of your mom is the right thing, then do it now no matter how hard it will be or how many sacrifices you have to make. God will make up for it." I really believe that. Try to focus on what's important.

Mr. Giovanni

Mr. Giovanni is a 57-year-old white marketing executive with a very businesslike manner. Immediately after greeting me at the door of his house, we sat down and he started the interview. He is an only child, and he and his wife returned from out West seven months ago to his hometown to care for his widowed 81-year-old mother. She has been diagnosed with multi-infarct dementia, and each series of strokes has left her more impaired, both physically and cognitively. He always knew that when the time came, he would take on the responsibility of caring for his mother. There was never any doubt of this commitment. Mr. Giovanni stated simply, "My mother has a need, and I will do it for my mother. I think there is a time and place when you do it. At least that's my feeling, and maybe my Catholic upbringing." Later in the interview, he further discussed this decision:

We were at the point where we had to make some commitments and help my mom, so we decided then—my wife and I—that her [his mother's] urgency was critical and was a priority, and we decided that we would move back. We would move back rather than move her to Colorado, because the doctors advised against that, the high altitude thing, which I am not sure is valid, but nevertheless. We said, "All right. We'll come back and walk her through the whole thing."

Mr. Giavonni was also very dissatisfied with the nursing home care his mother had been receiving, and decided that this was a time in his life when he could make a major life change. His own children were grown. They had finished college and were married. He stated:

We could afford to do this and we could say, "Well, okay. We could make that sacrifice." It didn't appear that the quality of life my mother was going to receive in a nursing home was good, and that was the thing that motivated us. We didn't feel that was the way we wanted her to live. We wanted to give her every opportunity to have as normal a life in as normal an environment as we could. So we sold my business and moved here.

Mr. Giovanni described his mother's present condition. She was in the later stage of dementia. She could transfer herself from her wheelchair to her bed with assistance, and she could sit up with his assistance. He is giving her total care. Like Mr. Florenzo and Mr. Rolinski, the other two men who also typify this "going the extra mile" type of caregiver, Mr. Giavonni is involved in the personal hands-on care for his mother. He discusses his caregiving role:

I'm her chief caregiver. We get up around eight o'clock and I lift her out of bed and put her on the toilet. Then we come in and have breakfast, take her back and give her a complete sponge bath and brush her teeth. Then I bring her into the living room or do some exercises, and in late morning she either watches some TV or dozes off. I clean things up and then it's time for lunch. We get her completely dressed after lunch, and she takes a late afternoon nap.

Mr. Giovanni has someone come in to watch his mother when he needs to go out to work. "But I'm with my mom seven days a week." He has a retired cousin living with them whom he can count on to help in an emergency as a companion for a short period of time, but the responsibility for his mother's care is solely on his shoulders.

Moving back home, he had to change professions. Because of his age and the downsizing in the marketing and sales job in his specialty, he was having difficulty finding work. He also needed a job that would allow him to work out of his house and schedule his own time, allowing for much flexibility. So, he started a new career in porcelain and formica repair, which, at the time of the interview, was just getting off the ground. He stated that with this new job, "My clients usually allow me my own time, so I can fit them into my caregiving schedule."

The Giovannis' relocation has also resulted in sacrifices to his wife's career. She had been working as an administrative assistant in various areas of the health care industry, from admitting to marketing. Finding a new job in this area was difficult, so she is now working in a farmers' market. As Mr. Giavonni said, "She's really the key figure. Without her cooperation and consent, none of this would be possible." But Mr. Giavonni is very sensitive and aware of the sacrifices he has asked his wife to make. He expressed his feelings about this:

The most difficult thing is the sacrifice that you have to . . . my wife . . . I just feel terrible about stealing these years from her because we are at an age. . . . This is not what we had planned for our mid-fifties. It wasn't the direction we were headed in, and I feel bad about stealing those from her. I hope that somewhere in the future we'll be able to make up for that some way or somehow. That's my biggest concern. That's the thing I really regret most. In the last seven months, we have been only able to steal away together for three or four dinners and a couple lunches. I mean, she understands. She's almost too good. I wish sometimes she would get angry with me and walk out, go away for a week, just for her own sanity.

He continued talking about how little time he has with his wife because of his responsibilities to his mother.

I'm really the only person that my mother relates to. I'm the only one that can calm her down—if she can be calmed down—when those crises hit. We have a sailboat. In fact, I've pulled it out of the marina and put it in storage because it looks like we're not going to use it in the near future. What I am asking her [his wife] to do is very, very difficult for a human relationship to endure.

Respite, time away from his caregiving duties, for now is out of the question for Mr. Giovanni. When he was younger, to get away and deal with various frustrations and stress in his life, he would use a punching bag or play golf; but not now.

There's no time to take a walk or play any golf. It's difficult to do things so far down on the priority list—you feel guilty doing it. Once in awhile

I can do it very early in the morning before my mother wakes up, but I would feel guilty doing it when I should be doing something else. Where if I ignored my mother, I wouldn't enjoy it because I'd be afraid that something would happen to her while I wasn't there. And I'd never forgive myself.

Accepting the caregiver role for his mother has changed Mr. Giovanni's entire life. It has changed his marital relationship, his career, and geographic location; it has also affected him on deeper levels, internally in terms of his personality and coping strategies, and also in his mother-son relationship. During our interview, he initiated the discussion about the changes he has seen in himself, including some positive ones. His business style of problem solving did not always work in his new role. He shared these reflections:

Initially we all try to operate in a certain way. Particularly if we do any type of management. So, we have a certain kind of process in which we approach things and we take a narrow vision of the thing. We kind of define the scope of what needs to be accomplished and go right at it; that's the way I always operated. We knew what the goal was, what we wanted to accomplish, and what we had to do to get there. I find now it's different. You have to play it by ear. You have to be versatile. You have to be extremely patient, very sensitive, and if you're not, I mean, the consequences are severely handicapping to you. That person becomes much more frustrated and much more difficult and it takes you much longer to do everything. In that way, I think I've become much more tolerant than I ever was raising our children, or even with my wife, or managing our own lives. You become extremely sensitive in that regard.

With further probing and reflection, he continued:

I guess what happened previously in my life was that in raising our own family, my wife was always there with the empathy, sympathy, and understanding. She was the shock cord and kept it all together. I could pop in, get a recap of the events, make a decision and pop out. It's kind of reversed itself now, because my wife has really been taken out of the scenario. I'm the only person my mother relates to.

Mr. Giovanni also described the changes in his relationship with his mother, which is very complex.

We've got a mother-son relationship and that's still a superior support relationship to some extent. In fact, I feel guilty sometimes when I know I should tell my mother some things. That may be applicable in the old relationship, but not in the new relationship; it's just you gotta change directions. Sometimes I've heard my mother use words I didn't know she knew. It's embarrassing. It's just shocking. If it's one of our children, we'd know intuitively how to handle it, but now it's my mother in a wheel-chair. And one of the most difficult things to deal with is she requires assistance to get in and out, and she fights me.

He continued with these thoughts about their relationship:

You experience a full range of emotions; sooner or later you will experi-ence all of them. My nature is to try to analyze things, to go back and lay there quietly and think "What happened?" "How did I react?" and "Boy, I don't want to do that again." Sometimes you need a drink; sometimes you feel sorry for yourself. You wanna die. Sometimes you sit there and you get a little mad at God and say, "I'd rather be in another place," but that usually doesn't last very long. Somewhere in the middle of this pe-riod you may start addressing her as an object rather than, that's your mother that person. It's difficult. And it's your mother. That's the person you love, and she is doing all these things.

Outside of the cooperation and support of his wife, Mr. Giovanni found limited support in his seven months of intense caregiving. The few sessions of support groups for caregivers that he attended did not fit his needs. Mr. Giovanni was seeking information; he was not interested in the emotional support of a support group. He stated:

Somehow or other, I didn't fit [in the support group]. I didn't get a lot of benefits from it. I couldn't. They were friendly people, don't get me wrong, but they seemed to have their own little agendas and in many cases they had husbands or spouses that had passed on and hung in to get to know these people and it was their extension—their extended family. That was nice, but in my case I was looking for things I needed. I needed a network of caregivers [to hire]. I needed to identify doctors. They were sympathetic, but couldn't point me in the right direction. I needed to get things done. You know what has to be done, but to find the right people, that's the very difficult thing in the whole process.

The role of the Church in his mother's illness has also been a disappointment for Mr. Giovanni, and has provided little assistance for his mother or himself.

My mother has been in this particular parish for 30 years. She's been in this area a long time and has contributed a lot of time and help and is very well respected. I called the pastor once about something, and he referred me to the yellow pages, if you can believe in News, that's not the way it used to be. It used to be, you talked with the pastor and the pastor said, "Okay, Jill, let me make a phone call for you and I'll get back to you." He'd make that connection with somebody and that person would call you back and you'd make the appointment and all of a sudden you had the right person, and this person could help you.

Living out of town for many years left him with few friends, and changing careers left him out the loop of joining the business associations he knew, where he might have discovered further sources of assistance.

I used to know a lot of people, but I haven't lived here for close to 30 years. That's quite a lapse in time. You're not the same. The relationship is not the same. It's still nice, but not the same. If I had stayed in my area, sales and marketing, that would have been a different story. There would have been organizations and things that I could have joined that would have often led to those connections.

Thus Mr. Giovanni has been left often to his own resourcefulness and perseverance. He developed some of his own basic equipment to help him care for his mother. He designed a new type of shower chair for her. He shared with pride his accomplishment:

To get a person from a wheelchair into a tub or shower situation, there aren't many things that can do that. And those chairs you sit in are not conducive for someone in my mother's condition. So, I improvised. I took a transfer bench and I took a chair, and I made a swivel chair out of it so she could sit with a seat belt and lift her leg up and just turn her in the thing. Now, she's got a secure device she can shower with.

Mr. Giovanni strongly felt that more of this type of equipment was needed. "Someone needs to develop and market this type of 'low-tech' equipment to help caregivers."

His parting advice to other sons taking on the caregiving role is a mixture of philosophy and fact. Mr. Giovanni expressed his thoughts this way:

The first advice I would give them is they should read the book The 36 Hour Day, because it [caring for a parent] is not what it appears to be. It's far more complicated than that; it's much deeper. Also they need to find a doctor they can talk to and trust and who will call them back. It takes a lot of stick-to-its. You have to really discipline yourself to accept some of the things that you're going to be addressing. It's hard. It's difficult. It's kind of a trial-by-error process. There's no guidelines.

Mr. Giovanni's, Mr. Polanski's, and Mr. Florenzo's narratives presented above illustrate the type of son caregiver who "goes the extra mile." Their narratives are filled with commitment, love for their parents, sacrifice, putting their "personal life on hold," and the provision of hands-on personal care to their parents in their homes. Like the husband caregivers, these three men made major lifestyle changes to care for their parents. Their parents' care took the first priority in their lives.

"The Strategic Planner"

Many of the sons used a problem-solving approach to aid them in caring for their ill parent and they often took charge of making key decisions. But this type of son, named "the strategic planner," did more than that. They were predominantly successful businessmen who tackled the care of their parents as they would any other project that they were managing. As one son stated, "I keep my father's folder on my desk, as I do all my projects, and pull it out and work on it for awhile every day." Their words and actions demonstrated an acceptance of the responsibility for caring for their ill parents, and also their management and planning strategies for providing that care. This was the predominant theme of their narratives. These sons logically sort out the steps and alternatives available to get their parents the kind of care that they need. This strategic-planning approach helps them take their well-honed management skills and use them to orient to the role of caregiver. Talk of their emotions was kept to a minimum. Most of the day-to-day personal care for the ill parent was provided by their well parent or paid caregivers. Mr. Malloy and Mr. Klein illustrate this type of son caregiver.

Mr. Malloy

Mr. Malloy is a tall, white, married, physically fit man in his early fifties with a demeanor that still shows traces of his former military background. He recently took advantage of an early retirement offer from his company to start his own business related to health care management. The interview took place in the office of his home, where he is now working.

He is one of three sons from a large family of seven siblings. His father is moving into the middle stage of Alzheimer's disease, but is still living at home with his wife and with much support from Mr. Malloy, the other children, and the grandchildren. It is a very supportive and devoted family; Mr. Malloy recently moved his parents to a location near him.

Soon after his father's diagnosis, Mr. Malloy became the main planner, responsible for his father's care. He had his mother write a memo to the other family members suggesting he take on this role because of his location and expertise. He discussed how this responsibility came about.

I suggested to my mother early on that because of my close proximity and because I knew how to access resources that she write a letter to the family suggesting that I do the facilitation. All my siblings suffer from the same frustration of how do we deal with this thing? How do we help Dad? They do what they can, but they have other things going on in their families. They don't have the accessibility that I have since I work out of my house or the knowledge; every day I can go over and see my parents.

Mr. Malloy is in the process of getting more services to assist his mother, who is reluctant to accept help.

I am in the process of modifying the bathroom and I've been attempting to hire a person to come and help bathe my father. There is a waiting list, and what I've done, I picked one intake screener at the agency and I leave her a message every two days. I say, "Hi, how are you today? I don't think you probably have had any change, but our need is still just as critical as it was before and I just want to give you an update." If we don't get some sort of response fairly quickly, then I have another possible person who can do it.

He is in the process of working with his mother "to bring her along" so she can see what needs to be done next.

I sat down with my mother and explained to her that we all have good intentions and people always say they are willing to do it, but without a regular routine that's done by someone outside the family, things won't ever get done. I'm trying to plot her along to make some decisions and once they're done, go on to the next one.

The issues down the road obviously are a nursing home with an Alzheimer's wing. How do we do that? How do we get on the waiting list? Whether they're willing to take that step? I think, though, it starts with me because I asked for the responsibility.

His parents have a friend who just entered an assisted-living facility, and Mr. Malloy has taken his mother for a visit to introduce her to the idea. He also took his father for a visit. With a family wedding out of town in a few months, he hopes to convince his mother that it might be best for his father to stay in that facility's short-stay respite care unit. Mr. Malloy said:

I plan on saying, "Well, Dad really can't travel out of town. We could put him in this facility for a brief respite for you." Like a trial basis, and that's kind of where I'm going. I think this respite plan would be a good way to have everybody [his siblings] look at it and start to see them [their parents] there. Then it becomes more palatable to start a discussion. If we all could see Dad in that environment, that could be step one, and then the financial thing is step two, and Mom could be step three.

Mr. Malloy has taken on the role of strategic planner to aid his parents and family in their attempts to deal with the disease. He is constantly planning and making decisions to move his family ahead and prepare them for the future. But he too sometimes has difficult times dealing with his father's illness. He admits that "it's pretty hard for anyone to see what my mother goes through on a day-to-day basis. It's very emotional for me; remember I am a junior [named after his father]."

He also has to manage working with his other siblings, who are often not as far along in the acceptance as he is with his father's illness, and they often approach the situation differently. He describes his relationship with his siblings regarding this situation.

The word "caregiver" is not the same for a son as it is for a daughter. My sisters are much more emotional about Dad. Not because they care more; it's just the nature of the person. Are we ever going to see eye-to-eye? Probably not. Men have a tendency to be very competitive and very matter-of-fact. Even my brother and I take two very different approaches.

Throughout this difficult time and conflict with his siblings, his wife has been his main source of support. She acts as his sounding board and safety valve when he needs to release some pressure. She has experience working with disabled children and their families, and understands this type of situation. He will often "bounce ideas off " his wife.

Yet with all this work and dedication, Mr. Malloy does not receive any satisfaction from his ability to help his parents. The bottom line has not changed. As he says:

I'm not satisfied when I don't see improvement. I think what satisfaction means to me is having done something that makes a difference, and maybe all those things would have made a difference if I were in a business situation or I had a profit margin, but when I look at it from a family standpoint it's neither satisfying or dissatisfying. I don't even know what would satisfy me. I guess I would be satisfied if my father could get better. Now my mother always has to thank me. For what? I didn't do anything. I might come over and shave him, but that didn't solve the problem.

His guidance to other caregivers reflects the value he places on planning ahead:

If it's diagnosed early on, you can start planning. You may need someone to look you straight in the eye and say, "Hey, look, you're not being rational with this disease. If you think it's going to be cured, it's not going to be cured." The earlier they arrive at that, the more realistic they can plan. I think not only for accepting the disease for what it is but for accepting that there are only limited resources.

Mr. Klein

I met with Mr. Klein soon after the death of his father. Although his father had been diagnosed with Alzheimer's disease only three years ago, he died unexpectedly of another illness. This white 46-year-old only child was in the midst of grieving for his father, and he was trying to come to terms with his loss, and with the "horrific" experience he had confronted as a caregiver of an Alzheimer's patient. Yet he insisted on doing this interview with the hope it might help other sons.

Even in the midst of this emotionally difficult time for Mr. Klein, his managerial approach to dealing with his father's care was evident. As he said, "I did the research, proposed the solution to the family, and then guided the decision, but the problem with this disease is there are no good answers." His mother provided the main hands-on care to his father until a nursing home became necessary.

Throughout this caregiving experience Mr. Klein was the one who was in charge, trying to make things happen, though he had much guidance and support from his wife, who is a social worker, and his close contacts with the local Alzheimer's Association. As he said, "I was still driving, but I was driving it with a lot of advice and counsel."

Mr. Klein immediately started the interview by dividing up his caregiving experience into three categories and evaluating each one. He described this experience:

I thought about this, and I tend to think in categories. For me there were three major categories: One was understanding the disease; another was understanding the system—the health care system, the provider system, the reimbursement system, all the system stuff that goes along with man-

aging the disease; and the third part was the managing of me and my family and how we were all feeling—the touchy feely piece of it.

The first part was the easiest for me; in some ways it was a research project. Like with my work, before you go out on a sales call you find out all you can about their business. And this was the part where there was the "most stuff" readily available. You can literally go to the medical library or get pamphlets from the association. That was the easy part.

For him, understanding "the system" and accessing it was the hard part.

The system didn't facilitate helping me try to get things under control. It absolutely exacerbates what a disease does to a family. I tried to speak to my family internist [to learn more about his father's other terminal illness] so I could guide the medication treatment if there was any, and make conscious decisions, knowledgeable decisions. And I would get answers like, "You don't have to worry about it." When he [his father] was transferred to the nursing home, I wanted to know if there were decisions we should be making about pain management. I just wanted to know, as part of the care and treatment of my father. And I would get a response, "Don't worry about this, we'll manage it. Why do you want to know?" And I said, "Because we have financial decisions to make. We have care decisions to make. We have living wills and all those decisions to make." I mean the whole thing just beats the family up terribly, the not knowing, the having to run around to talk to the social workers to try to access the system. And I have a full-time job. I have to travel extensively. I was doing a lot of this over the phone long distance.

In response to a question about the third piece, the emotional piece, Mr. Klein responded simply but poignantly: "I wanted to hold my father's hand and go through this last phase with him. And they really didn't let you. You know, the system didn't let you. You had to fight for whatever time you could get."

When asked how it was decided that he would take this active managerial role, Mr. Klein thought for a minute and then said:

I don't think it was decided. I think I'm just pushy. It seemed like a management project, and I manage projects. And so I said, "I'll do this.

I'll do this and you do that." And still being sensitive to the role she [his mother] wanted to play and needed to play. I wanted to do more to alleviate her of the burnout and those kind of things. Periodically, my wife would say something like, "Do you know how your mother's feeling?" So, I'd go talk with her.

Yet, even with all his effort to help his mother and his father, he didn't feel he had done enough. As he said, he tries to "operate out of a principle of fairness," and he feels he did not shoulder his amount of the responsibility. And his father's situation could have been worse. Mr. Klein admitted:

There never was enough time to do what I felt I should have done. I let my mother carry too much of it because she is strong. She picked up the slack. I should have picked up more of the slack. And I sit here and sound like, gee, I've had this tough time. I mean I've seen what other people who have dealt with this disease for 10 years. They had loved ones who didn't know them and screamed. You know I've looked down that abyss and thankfully I didn't have to go down it.

Mr. Klein ended the interview with some suggestions for health care professionals. What would have been most helpful to him would be a list of 20 "do's" and "don'ts" about giving the care, understanding the disease, and working the system. He said angrily:

You ought not to have to go through this hodge-podge out there and try to piece it together yourself. It ought to be—here is step one and here are your choices. I'd like the professionals to come together and fill the void. I'd like them to say "Okay, for this terrible disease called Alzheimer's there are phases. Phase one looks like this, and here are some of the options available as you cope with phase one," and the same for phase two and phase three. But the consumer, who is generally the person who needs help, has to piece all of that together at a time when it's the last thing they want to be doing.

Both Mr. Klein and Mr. Malloy illustrate the characteristics of this type of son described as "the strategic planners." They used their managerial skills to adapt to their role as caregivers as they tried to plan and direct their parents' care. Their parents' care became a very special project for them to oversee, but with an emotional component that was often hard for them to manage. They were committed to caring for their parents and felt deeply for them, and used their business skills to aid their parents to the utmost of their abilities.

"Sharing the Care"

The last type of son caregiver provided care to an ill parent as a team with help from a wife or a sibling. Sometimes they provided hands-on care and sometimes supportive care. The two people were equal partners in the provision of care and the decision making. Often each brought a different perspective and set of skills to the caregiving experience. Most often the son brought that "partner" with him to the interview. They comfortably answered the questions together, sometimes completing the other person's thoughts. Each person was aware of and acknowledged the contribution their "partner" made to the caring of the ill parent and often well spouse. Mr. Ford, the O'Casey brothers, and Mr. Irvine typify this type of son caregiver.

Mr. and Mrs. Ford

The interview with Mr. and Mrs. Ford took place over lunch at a local restaurant one Saturday afternoon. They are a warm, caring, unassuming couple. He works as a para–health care professional. They are in their late thirties and have two young children. He is the middle child of three siblings; his brother, the oldest child, lives out of town, and his younger sister lives locally.

Mr. Ford's mother was diagnosed a year ago with Alzheimer's disease. Though she is still able to maintain the household for her husband and herself, she is beginning to have more difficulty with household chores, especially cooking. Mr. Ford's sister is having difficulty accepting her mother's diagnosis, and still denies anything is wrong. Thus, Mr. Ford and his wife are the main sources of support for his parents. He went with his parents to a support group designed for early diagnosed individuals and their families that met for eight weeks.

While describing his mother's illness, they discussed the difficulty they have had accepting it, and how painful it is for them to see this happen to someone they love. Mr. Ford has trouble expressing his thoughts and emotions, so his wife often gets him started. Mrs. Ford said:

When you have a mom like her—I mean, she's a super person. Everything was perfect. She had a perfect house. She could cook out of this world. Always busy, always active, and then all of sudden there are so many things she just can't do. And she is young to me [63 years old]. And you say, "No, that just can't be." You try to push it out of your mind. I've known this family since I was 16. It's very difficult.

Mr. Ford continued, admitting, "See, all of this brings out emotions and feelings that have never been brought out in our family, especially by Mother and Dad." Mrs. Ford added, "They showed their love in many ways, but they just never said the words or showed any affection." Mr. Ford confessed, "Yes. I find it easier to do with other people, and my wife is a good role model." His wife taught him to open up and share his feelings. She comes from a family where open communication comes naturally.

One of the major supportive roles that Mr. Ford provides for his parents is transportation. They live in a rural area, and his father no longer likes to drive at night or for long distances, so Mr. Ford will take either his mother or both his parents to meetings in the city an hour away. He describes one of the trips:

She [his mother] misses those people [from the support group] so she wanted to go to that meeting in town, but she knew my dad didn't want to drive up there. And all of a sudden she starts to crying. I didn't know what it was until I realized. So, I told her, "Well, we're going to go. We'll go to the meeting. I'll be over to pick you up. So, if Dad doesn't want to go, he doesn't have to go. We'll go."

Mrs. Ford views her role with her parents-in-law as a source of support they can depend on. For her mother-in-law she said, "I feel like I'm looking out for her in a way. Like, when we're together, I don't want her to feel uncomfortable or feel like she can't do anything. I try to help her discreetly. I try not to make a big deal out of it." For her father-in-law, "I just want him to know I am here. Gosh, I've been part of this family for 20-some years and I just want him to know I love him a lot and I want to be there for them."

Mr. and Mrs. Ford jointly discussed the role in caring for their parents that his older brother, who lives out of town, plays. Mr. Ford said, "He talks to them on the phone quite a bit. He communicates more with them than I do." Mrs. Ford chimed in, "He was the first one to really say, 'We need to do something about Mom.' We see her every day, and it was a few months since he had come home, and could see the difference. He called you [Mr. Ford] up at work and said, 'Let's do something.' He initiated getting the diagnosis."

Even in their advice to other sons involved in caring for a parent with dementia, Mr. and Mr. Ford shared similar suggestions. Mrs. Ford said, "Just be there for them. Don't be overbearing or try to take over; but just be there for the love and support that they need." Mr. Ford added, "That's basically it. What my wife says is very true. You need to tell them 'I'll be there for you when the time comes,' because it's a long process and everybody needs help sometimes."

Mr. and Mrs. Ford worked as a team, "sharing the care," with each contributing according to their ability. They are both equally committed to helping Mr. Ford's parents and are actively participating in the care.

The O'Casey Brothers

Joseph and John O'Casey arrive at the interview together, though it was Joseph who initiated the contact. These men are the oldest of six siblings, and are the most involved in their father's care. Joseph O'Casey is the oldest son and readily accepts his responsibility because of that status. Their father is in the late stage of Alzheimer's disease, and their stepmother has reached a point where she can no longer care for him; he is now in a nursing home. Both sons were supportive of this decision and encouraged their stepmother to make this move.

The two sons' personalities and looks complement each other. Joseph O'Casey is tall, slender, quiet, and quite serious. He handles some of his father's financial and legal matters. John is shorter, heavier, more boisterous and gregarious than his brother, and has a good sense of humor. He handles more of the emotional and personal needs of his father and stepmother. He could also express for his brother what they were both feeling. Together they made a good partnership.

As Joseph said at the outset of the interview:

My brother and I are the oldest of six children, five boys and a girl, and we are probably the ones who see my Dad the most often. Some children live out of town and others are having difficulty dealing with the whole situation. We understand this and are not keeping score.

John chimed in:

To be honest with you, I didn't know if I would be able to handle it either. I've been doing things I didn't think I'd ever do for him of a personal nature, like trying to put his teeth in so he can eat. But it was tough for both of us because, "This is my dad. I have to do these things for him." And you'd sit there and maybe cry for awhile.

In describing the role each man played in convincing their step-mother she could no longer care for their father, their different functions became evident. Joseph talked about the financial and legal ramifications, and John talked about the socioemotional aspects. Thinking back to that time over a year ago, Joseph said, "There was the financial thing, I do my dad's taxes, and luckily we put her in touch with this attorney. Later I wrote a letter to the attorney saying, 'I appreciate the help you gave her.'"

John expressed the concern that caring for their father was too much for her and that she could not continue giving him the total 24-hour care he was beginning to need. He added, "I talked to her [their stepmother] and said:

"He [their father] needs 24-hour care and you can't give it to him. We're worried about you right now. You're in good shape. You pride yourself on the way you take care of yourself, and you're gonna go downhill real fast. That's a disservice to yourself and your children to allow yourself to go downhill like that. We can't let you do that anymore." I really talked to her and said, "You just can't do it. You got to face the facts."

Joseph continued, "So we felt that despite her complaints about the cost, we achieved our end by getting this attorney involved too." John interrupted, adding, "We achieved our end because we think we saved her from herself." Joseph interrupted and said, "Something might have happened to her." And John added, "And I think it would have."

The two sons were very comfortable talking with each other about their father's situation, often completing and adding to each other's sentences. They each appreciated the role the other son played and used the word "we" throughout their narrative as demonstrated in the dialogue above.

Even when talking about what helped them cope through this difficult time, the theme of sharing the care and how they rely on each other is evident. Joseph said, "I think the fact that we are together, we're always together, and I think it's helped us. I think we probably talk more now than we ever did." John added, "Our mother died [25 years ago] and we all went about our own way." Joseph concluded, "Well, when your mother dies, the anchor of the family home is gone."

In their advice to future son caregivers, again their different roles in the caregiving process are expressed. Joseph O'Casey said, "Try to understand the financial aspects of this. It's not necessarily something that will deplete somebody's assets. And I would definitely recommend getting legal counsel." John O'Casey's advice was, "I would encourage people who are definitely going to be faced down the road with a nursing home to start checking them out right now. Talk to people that have had relatives in nursing homes and just find out what the problems are, and get accustomed to the idea."

Mr. Irvine's narrative, presented below, also illustrates well the type of son who "shared the care."

Mr. Irvine

I had met Mr. Irvine and his wife a number of times, as we worked together on committees for the Alzheimer's Association. As a matter of fact, he is one of the sons who strongly urged me to do research on son caregivers because he felt they were always being forgotten. He is a tall African-American man in his late fifties with a quick wit, a wonderful sense of humor, and a panache for telling stories. He has held a number of jobs over the course of his life from security guard at a large corporate headquarters to owning a men's clothing store. His mother had died a year earlier of Alzheimer's disease. The narrative of this couple's caregiving experience blends together his humor, his philosophy on life, and his love for his mother. We met for the interview without his wife, but the important role she played in his mother's care was the cornerstone of his narrative.

Mr. Irvine is an only child, and as his mother's disease became progressively worse, he brought her from her home in the South to live with him and his wife. This was not an easy decision for him. He said, "My mother had told me straight out, 'Son, if you take me away, I'll be dead in a couple of months because I just can't stand leaving my home.' I had a grave responsibility." But he had made a promise as a child years ago to her that he would care for her, and he was determined to honor that commitment out of duty and a deep sense of love.

His father had died in a car accident a number of years ago. He had since heard from many of his mother's neighbors and his child-hood friends that his mother's behavior had became "quite strange," which was very disconcerting for him because his mother was al-ways a very pleasant and kind woman. During his frequent trips to visit her, he had not observed this behavior. Mr. Irvine said, "I prayed to God that he would give me the sign and the information that I would need to know when to go and get her." After a potentially life-threatening incident happened to his mother, he knew he could not delay moving her any longer.

This led to a poignant but humorous story about moving his mother and their drive back to Cleveland. He told the story:

I got a call from a friend in Alabama saying she [his mother] was pack-ing her car with a few incidentals and a pistol that I had given her for her protection, and that she was going home. She didn't recognize her own house. But fortunately for me, one of my schoolmates lived right next door to our family home. They really guarded her for me. So when he saw this occurring, he sneaked over to the house and unplugged one of the wires on the car so she couldn't get the car started. But my mom was sharp enough at the time to know that she keeps her car at the shop and the only reason it wouldn't start was because someone had been messing with it. So, when she saw my friend there, she went after him, screaming and cussin' at him, chasing him through the front door of the neighbor's house and right out the back door. Here's this 70-year-old lady chasing this big guy around the house. I bet it was hilarious, my mother running right behind him. Then they called me, and I said if they could contain her till morning, I would catch the midnight flight out and be there by 7:00 in the morning. When I got there in the morning, she didn't remember anything about the occurrence. We then started our ride back to Cleveland.

I loaded her car up with her clothes and we drove back to Cleveland. Things were fine till we got close to home and she saw a sign that said Cleveland. She started cussing and carrying on; and I'm irritable because I had been driving. Now, it's a 10- or 11-hour drive and I had no sleep, and I just lost it. I said, "Damnit Mother! If you don't shut up!" She pulled herself up in her seat and said in that voice, "I can remember a time when kids respected their elders!" I knew I had better be quiet and thought, "The Lord's gonna get me now." So, I just rolled the window down and started, "woo woo woo," blowing out the window, just trying to get control of my faculties. But the closer I got to Cleveland, the more agitated she got. She finally said, "If I had wanted to come to Cleveland, I would have drove my own damn car."

When I got to town, I pulled my car into my fiancée's driveway [Mr. Irvine and his wife were at that point engaged to be married]. I got out of the car and told her, "My mother's outside. If you want her, go get her, because she is driving me crazy. I cannot stand it. I got to go home and get some sleep." She took her out of the car. She kept her that night for me.

Mr. Irvine reflects back on the role his wife has played in caring for his mother ever since she arrived on her doorstep in Cleveland: "The relationship with my wife-to-be up to this present time has been one of two people coming together and shouldering the responsibility. When I am not at my best, my wife is." He continued thinking, "It's like having an alternator on your car to take care of the pressure when the battery is getting low. Once you get it started, now you got to keep it running. That's the effect my wife has on me." When he was feeling the stresses of caregiving, his wife was there to calm him down, and to take her turn providing him the needed relief.

His wife-to-be made the trip down South with Mr. Irvine to help them pack up his mother's house. Mr. Irvine commented:

She worked tirelessly with me and my mom, because my mom determined we were going to bring every piece of everything she had or she wasn't coming. I had to rent the biggest truck that you could imagine. And I thought, my God, what I am going to do with all this stuff. My house is not that big. So after talking with my wife-to-be, I ended up putting some of my furniture in her house and put my mother's furniture into my house. Slowly I would bring my furniture back and take some of my mother's furniture and put it into the basement and give some away. Those were rough times, really rough times. The thing that got me through it was the fact that I'm very spiritual; and my wife, for if it had not been for her, I wouldn't have survived.

Mr. Irvine's mother lived with them until her death, and both he and his wife took turns caring for her. Owning his own store provided him with the flexible hours that were essential as he took his turns caring for his mother; his wife worked also. If he needed to close his store for a few hours to be available for his mother, he would. However, it was the constant support from his wife, both physically and emotionally, his deep spiritual beliefs, and his sense of humor that helped him to cope.

Mr. Irvine commented about his strong religious beliefs: "Everyone needs to believe in something. That's my personal feeling, and for me it's God. I don't make any moves until I find out from him if this is what I need to do. It always works for me."

Laughter also provided a coping mechanism for Mr. Irvine and his wife, and his humor often helped them keep things in perspective. Mr. Irvine stated:

I've always had a good sense of humor. I have a knack for that. I got that sense of humor from my mother. It has always paid to laugh when you find yourself in a situation for which you cannot come up with a solution. If you get frustrated and all worked up, to laugh gives you an opportunity to be free. It's like putting your car in neutral. You don't have to worry where you are going any more.

Mr. Irvine knew that they were giving the best possible care to his mother, which also provided him with a sense of satisfaction and helped him through some of the difficult times. He revealed,

You see what this caregiving did for me is to prevent what happens to other folks when they are screaming and hollering and carrying on at funerals, and they weren't there when their parents needed them. My mother died and I had no guilt. My mother died in peace, so I have peace with her going because I knew that everything that was humanly possible was secured for my mother.

Mr. Irvine had two suggestions for other son caregivers. His first suggestion had to do with communications. He reflected:

The one thing a son really needs is to learn how to communicate and that would help them out with their wives. Men don't talk, and that's a real crisis. It's a crisis in their lives even without somebody being sick. So they go into this [caregiving] with no talking skills, and they're not able to verbalize. I think that's what they need up front is really some skills in verbalization with women, which would make life better for them all the way around.

His other suggestion is that sons should not be afraid to ask for help, and particularly to seek the support of their local Alzheimer's Association. Mr. Irvine commented:

We need to have somebody there with open arms saying, "I understand what you are going through. I'm here for you." That's what this organization [the Alzheimer's Association] here has done for me. I've tried, as a result of what they've done for me, to loan myself to others in that process. Because, especially in the black community, people have had to fend for themselves for so long. I'll tell you, I've seen a lot of people almost lose it simply because they didn't know where to turn and what to do about the situation.

The Irvines, the O'Caseys, and the Fords personify this final type of son caregiver who is "sharing the care," be it with a wife or a sibling. Each partner in the caregiving brings his or her own perspective and unique set of skills to the experience, and each is committed to caring for an ill parent or parent-in-law with dementia.

Conclusions

This chapter described a topology of son caregivers, four different ways the 30 sons oriented themselves to their caregiving role. We designated the four groups as "the dutiful son," "going the extra mile," "the strategic planner," and "sharing the care." Each group has some unique characteristics that differentiate it from the other types.

The sons who constituted "the dutiful son" type discussed and emphasized their strong sense of duty toward their parents, and this was the central theme of their narratives. They used words and actions that expressed an obligation and sense of responsibility, and they were able to integrate this duty into their present lifestyle. Some sons expressed in their narratives much love and devotion for their parents, and others expressed more acceptance of this as what you do as a son. This type of son caregiver constitutes the largest portion of the sample for this study.

The "going the extra mile" type of son caregiver demonstrated a willingness to make complete lifestyle changes to care for their ill parents, changes that entailed bringing their parents into their own homes or moving into theirs, providing hands-on care, and much personal sacrifice. In essence, they took on the role of a "committed spouse caregiver" and encountered similar experiences such as social isolation, putting their personal lives on hold, and much caregiver burden and stress, which they were willing to voice. Their love for their parents, combined with a sense of duty and guilt, provided motivation for adaptation to this role. This was the central theme of their narratives.

The third way a group of sons oriented to their caregiving role was by using the management and planning skills they had learned in their world of work. These were "the strategic planners." The dominant theme of their narratives focused on their strategies and plans for seeking out and obtaining the needed care for their ill parents. They took charge, and their words and actions demonstrated this theme. Their parents' care became a special type of project for them to oversee, but included an overriding emotional component, which was often difficult for them to discuss. They too were deeply committed to caring for their parents.

The last type of son caregivers were the sons who "shared the care" of an ill parent as a team with a wife or a sibling, and adapted in this way to their role as son caregiver. This sharing provided them the strength, ability, and motivation to provide the care. It was the focal point of their narratives. Sometimes this partnership consisted of hands-on care, and at other times, because a well parent was providing that care, they provided supportive services. They were equal partners in the provision of care and decision making. Often each member of the partnership brought a complementary skill and perspective to the caregiving experience.

The sons interviewed tended to fall into one of these four types, though that did not mean there were not some overlapping characteristics. Listening to the words and actions of the narratives provided the clues to the predominant way a son oriented to his caregiving role and how they coped.

As the title of this chapter, "Toward a Typology of Son Caregivers" suggests, what is presented here is only a beginning attempt to understand how sons adapt to a role that is usually foreign to them. Thirty sons took on the role of caregiver to a parent with dementia and oriented to this responsibility in ways that were meaningful to them, and this guided them in their tasks. Much more research needs to be done to further our knowledge and understanding of how sons adapt to this role.

Chapter Seven
Sons
Service Implications—What Can We Learn?

Across the four types of caregivers, sons have consistent program and service suggestions irrespective of the approach taken to caregiving. In general, sons did not want social support programs, but preferred educationally oriented services. They wanted information about dementia and what impact it had on their parents' behavior, and how to access needed services. These men did not want to focus on their own emotional needs, nor to hear about others' situations. Several sons specifically stated they were not interested in "support group" type dementia programs. If a program was billed as an "educational program" they would be much more likely to attend. These sons wanted information that would help them in their decision-making process and then support and validate them in acting on these decisions.

The programs and services described here reflect this education/information-gathering orientation. What is presented in this chapter is a combination of the specific suggestions from the sons as well as our recommendations of possible programs that could meet their stated needs. These programs break down into four general areas: information, care management, support, and respite.

Information
The sons in our study consistently spoke about their need for information. They wanted to understand the basics about the disease as well as understand the workings of the service-delivery system. Sons were most often the information gatherers in their families, whether or not they provided the hands-on care to their parent. They wanted to understand the problem at hand and the possible solutions. This was consistent with the "taking charge" theme discussed in the pre-

vious chapter, and it was particularly true of the type of sons we've grouped as "the strategic planners." These sons handled their parents' care as they would other projects that they managed. They needed to learn thoroughly learn and "research" the situation before mapping out their plan.

The following are specific areas in which sons wanted information to assist them in their caregiving roles.

Information About the Disease

Almost across the board, the sons interviewed had received information about dementia, mainly from the Alzheimer's Association, an Alzheimer's research center, or their parent's physician. They said that this information was clear and helpful. Most of their frustration came from discovering what science and medicine still did not know about the disease. The sons wanted more answers about the cause of the disease and were frustrated to learn that finding a cure might still be decades away. Like many caregivers, the more they learned about Alzheimer's disease the more unanswered questions they had.

Sons want to be directed to resources where they can continue to get accurate, updated information on Alzheimer's. It is important to refer sons to agencies that can supply updated information, such as the Alzheimer's Association, Alzheimer's research centers, and the Alzheimer's Disease Educational and Referral Center of the National Institute on Aging, which provide newsletters and research updates on the disease. These newsletters help these sons stay in touch with the accurate information that they seek. Information from these organizations is also available on the Internet, through the World Wide Web, by doing a search using the keyword "Alzheimer's disease" (see also Appendix D for another option). Professionals should also be aware of which local libraries have specialized sections on dementia and refer sons to these.

One-time workshops, particularly those held in the evenings or on weekends, are likely to appeal to these men. These workshops do not require an ongoing time commitment, nor do they try to "support" those in the caregiving role. The men who attended such sessions viewed them as a place to hear an informed speaker, get some questions answered, and pick up literature that they could read at a later time.

Information about Community Resources, Service Delivery, and Service Evaluation

Sons clearly and consistently voiced their frustration with the lack of information on resources available in their community to assist them in the care of their parent. Many sons wanted to understand the different types of services available. They often found the service-delivery system a confusing web, a place where one professional referred you to another professional and then to a third without getting any clear answers. Suggestions these men gave for decreasing this confusion included providing them with a glossary defining common health care and social service terminology. They felt they spent too much time trying to figure out the difference between personal care aides and homemakers, or what was meant by assisted living versus skilled care. If they had a simple tool for understanding what these terms meant, it would allow them to make decisions more quickly on what they might find most useful. Another suggestion was the creation of a central intake or screening service knowledgeable in services for the elderly and those with dementia. This type of service would eliminate or reduce the frustration these men experienced in trying to find the appropriate service provider. This service should be well publicized so that a first-time user would be aware of its existence.

Sons suggested another area needing improvement was information on how to evaluate the quality of a service. Once they decided what service they wanted, for example, adult day care, they then wanted to know how to tell which were the good day care providers. Since providing caregiving services was usually an area that was relatively new to these men, they didn't immediately have the knowledge to be able to formulate questions that would help them to evaluate the quality of service. This lack of knowledge made some of these men uncomfortable and at times angry. They, as a group, consistently requested information that would help them understand more thoroughly the service and how it is delivered so they could emerge as educated consumers who could question and find the right match for their parent. Some of the questions these men wanted answered were:

- How do you determine if you are getting a high standard of care?
- What indicators of quality care can be used to evaluate these

services?
- What constitutes good home care?
- What constitutes good residential facilities?

These men specifically want a checklist of questions they should ask in evaluating the quality of services such as adult day care and nursing homes (see Appendices F and G).

Information About Equipment and Adaptive Devices
Many of the sons in our study were interested in learning more about equipment and adaptive devices that might assist in the tasks of caregiving such as bathroom safety rails, door locks, and identification bracelets for wanderers. Some sons had devised their own adaptive devices. The sons particularly wanted more information on how to determine what specifically would help their parent. Several men suggested a need for more organized and comprehensive information on the range and availability of adaptive equipment. Their questions included:

- How do you determine what devices are appropriate for the person with Alzheimer's?
- Where do you purchase these devices?
- How do you monitor the safety and effectiveness of these devices?

A workshop on this topic would provide the appropriate forum for answering these questions and be of much assistance to these son caregivers.

Financial and Legal Information
Caregiving sons were very involved in the financial matters of their parents. Sons expressed concerns about the cost of long-term care and the legal implications of making major medical decisions for a parent. Sons wanted information on Medicare, Medicaid, local assistance programs, power of attorney, and living wills. Workshops and literature on these topics held great interest for these men.

Information and Education in the Workplace
Sons, for the most part, did not discuss their feelings about caregiving

with their co-workers. Even though they didn't seek support from colleagues, they did express that it would be helpful if their boss or co-workers understood the demands that caregiving entails. A boss who does not understand that a worker has to leave the office suddenly because he receives a call saying that his parent was found wandering in the street puts additional stress on the caregiving son. An educated boss and co-workers can give the caregiver a degree of understanding that might relieve some of the embarrassment and pressure that many of the sons were feeling.

Information on Alzheimer's disease could be shared in the workplace through "lunch and learn" series, retirement planning sessions, and the distribution of literature. Information could also be made available through sessions with EAP (Employee Assistance Program) counselors.

Care Management

Without any previous caregiving history, sons often found themselves in the midst of the enormous tasks of taking over the management of their parents' every need. Sons, like most other caregivers, found themselves dealing with a health care system and social service system that was confusing, expensive, and difficult to access. In addition, sons were often holding down full-time jobs and struggling to continue their day-to-day lives while overseeing the increasing needs of someone with progressive dementia. Without using the actual words of case or care management, the sons in our study repeatedly described the need for this type of help.

The sons wanted help in their caregiving role and expressed the need for individualized professional advice in the care and management of their parent. They wanted a social worker or other professional to meet with them, possibly with other family members as well, and discuss in detail their caregiving circumstances. From this meeting sons wanted a how-to guide—something that would describe for them the type of care their parent needed, outline what types of services would be helpful at this point in time, where to go for these services, who to call (with names and phone numbers), and how to plan for the future. Sons said they particularly said they wanted to know about residential facilities, where to find a good nursing home, and how to get their parent admitted. Other sons wanted specific input on home adaptive equipment that would be helpful in their particular situation. They wanted to present the problem to the professional, and have the professional tell them how and where to go for the solution.

Some of the men in our study had contact with an individualized care management program that addressed many of these needs (see Appendix H). The attributes of this care management program that was most helpful to these men were:

- The individualized nature of the program: The social worker met to evaluate and discuss the particular problems and concerns of the client family.

- The flexibility of the program: The social worker arranged to meet with the family at a time that was convenient to the client. This was particularly helpful to working sons; meetings were able to be arranged in the evenings or on weekends. The social worker was also willing to come to the home or any other site that was most convenient to the son or other family members.

- The creation of a specific individualized plan: After lengthy discussions with the caregiving sons and others involved, the family was left with a written plan that detailed the strengths of their situation, the immediate problems, and a list of tasks that needed to be done to help alleviate some of these problems. This task list was very focused and specific. Task lists often included agencies (such as two or three home health agencies to call for help with personal care), services (such as the telephone number to call to order an ID bracelet for the parent who was wandering), as well as informal task delegation (such as sister Sue will come in on Tuesday evenings to relieve her brother of caregiving tasks for four hours). This individualized written plan came close to the type of step-by-step how-to guide many of the sons said they yearned for.

The need for this type of service speaks to the individualized need for help that the sons in our study repeatedly requested. They were not interested in generalized programs geared to the masses. Their time was at a premium, and they were not seeking support from others; they wanted the bottom line on how best to help their parent in their situation. Development of this personalized care management service with a written task list was one way to meet this need.

Support

Sons, in general, did not have strong friendship networks. Many confided in their wives or girlfriends, but aside from this limited network, they did not have an outlet for the multitude of feelings they had about their caregiving situation, including feelings of grief, confusion, frustration, and anger. Even when a supportive wife was present these men were reluctant to burden them with their intense feelings. Sons expressed concern because they were already splitting time between their wives, children, and the growing needs of their parents. In the interviews many expressed feelings of guilt, concerned that the care of their parent was pulling them away from quality time with their own families, yet they were reluctant to express these feelings to their wives or children.

Also, many sons expressed the fact that work was an escape, a place where they could forget about their caregiving concerns and bury themselves in the tasks at hand. It was not the place where they shared emotions with others.

Hence, this emotional isolation took its toll on some of the men interviewed. For some, the actual interview for the study was the first time these sons had discussed their intense feelings about their situation. Many expressed relief at having done so, and acknowledged a need for having a safe place to do this again. The sons who expressed a need for more emotional support specifically stated they would not feel comfortable doing so in a situation that mixed caregiving spouses with adult children. They wanted only wanted to talk with others of their generation (30–50 years old) who were caring for a parent. However, when presented with the option of meeting with other adult children, caregiver sons still expressed some reluctance in attending support groups.

A computer network as described in Chapter 4 and Appendix D seems to be a way that sons could connect with one another. This sample of sons had not accessed this mode of support, so it is difficult to make generalizations about its usefulness to this population.

Based on the expressed needs and issues of these sons, we recommend that a separate bulletin board for caregiving sons be established as a subsection of a telecomputing Alzheimer's support network. The anonymity, accessibility, and convenience of this type of support might prove to be a helpful link for these men.

Respite

Sons, like the husbands, consistently said that they needed more affordable, flexible, high-quality respite services. As previously noted, sons often used in-home or adult day care services for their parents with dementia. Many of the sons in this study were working, and many more were living in residences apart from their parents. Because they themselves were not live-in caregivers, the availability of respite services was a critical issue in whether or not they could keep their parent living in the community.

Sons reported that they desired adult day care services that were user-friendly to working people. This meant that day care hours should extend beyond nine to five, thus allowing working people to drop their relatives off on their way to the job and pick them up after they themselves got off work. Many of the sons longed for a day care service that was available on weekends and in the evenings. This type of service would truly be a respite to them, since the weekday service allowed them to go only to their jobs. It did not necessarily function as a true break from their routine of caregiving.

Sons reported problems when they needed to go out of town for business, or if they went on an occasional vacation with their family. They found very few affordable options for extended 24-hour respite. Although some nursing homes do provide this type of care, the cost for many of the sons in our study was prohibitive.

Service Implications: Contrasts between Husbands and Sons

In comparing the service recommendations of caregiving husbands and sons, it becomes clear that there are many similarities, and also striking contrasts. Both husbands and sons wanted information about the disease, caregiver education, information on how to hire help, and more flexible and affordable respite services.

In general, husbands expressed more emotional needs than did the sons. The disease disrupted the entire lifestyle of husbands, and they were seeking services that would help them adjust to this change. Husbands wanted to talk to other men in similar situations, and they wanted to understand how others dealt with this new phase of their life. They grieved for their losses and for their spouse. Husbands, like sons, expressed a need for information and educational programs, but husbands wanted more on the how-to's of hands-on personal care, while sons wanted information on navigating the service-delivery system.

Sons saw caregiving as a temporary task that they wanted to do well and efficiently, but knew that once completed, their lives would resume as before. They wanted to know where they could get good quality help that they could supervise to be sure their parents were well taken care of. Sons were less concerned with their own personal well-being than they were with seeing their parents through this difficult time.

As more men enter into caregiving roles, there will be an increasing need to provide service to this population. We feel it is essential to understand the needs of these men, their similarities and differences, so that a service system that is truly helpful will be developed.

Conclusions

Consistent with their problem-solving approach, sons wanted clear, concise information about the disease, what to expect, and the care options. They were not interested in supportive services or spending time discussing their feelings. They wanted to go right to the bottom line in the most direct and efficient manner. Their suggestions for improved services reflect this orientation. Information services including a dementia-specific referral system should be well publicized and user-friendly. Care management services should be flexible and highly individualized. Glossaries and checklists should be clear, precise, and readily available. Respite services should meet the needs of the working caregiver. Currently, these men feel isolated from others and the service-delivery system. If implemented, these service suggestions have the potential of meeting the expressed needs of these son caregivers, helping them to feel more a part of the system rather than outside of it, and ultimately aiding the son caregiver as well as the impaired parent.

Chapter Eight
Contrasts, Questions, and Final Reflections

With this concluding chapter, we bring together the narratives of the husbands and sons we interviewed. We compare their similarities and differences, summarize the findings, and pose some of the questions that still need to be answered about these and other male caregivers. Finally, we return to our original research questions and offer our closing reflections on this group of husbands and sons.

The limitations of this study are many. The information is based on narratives from 60 men who have accepted their responsibility for caring for a relative with dementia and who were willing to tell their stories. They are not representative of all the husbands and sons dealing with the devastating impact of dementia on a family member. In fact, these men in the study may be a unique group; more research on the growing population of male caregivers may or may not substantiate this possibility. Yet from the reflections of these husbands and sons emerges a more in-depth, diverse, and complex picture of the issues and struggles a man can have in his effort to provide care than has been previously reported. And thus, consequent upon these men's reflections, our knowledge and understanding of the male caregiving experience is enhanced.

Contrasts
Husbands and Sons
Originally when we conceived the idea for this research, both husbands and sons were chosen as the subjects, as we thought that as male caregivers they would have many issues and concerns in common, with only a few differences. In the course of the research, however, it became clear that there were many unanticipated differences, which are discussed below. The most prevalent similarity between

the husbands and sons in this study is their overriding sense of commitment and duty to care for their ill family members. They accepted this responsibility as "theirs," an acceptance that for many came with great emotional, social, and financial costs.

Both groups often used a problem-solving approach as they learned the new roles and tasks that fashioned them into caregivers and added another facet to their identities. They felt comfortable taking control of or supervising their relatives' care. It was a natural extension of their male role in our society. But the similarities between sons and husbands were sometimes overshadowed by the differences.

The husbands' lives were profoundly and deeply altered by their wives' illness. The sense of utter loss in their lives was clearly evidenced in their narratives. As a husband, quoted in Chapter 2, so astutely concluded about his situation, "I realized my life was changed forever . . . [and] I began the first day of the rest of my life."

The sons' reactions to their parents' illness was much more complex and contradictory. Although the sons were emotionally involved in the caregiving experience, they evidenced less overall intensity of emotion than the husbands. They were able to approach the caregiving more objectively and accept it more quickly than the husbands. As horrendous as the situation was, their lives would not be forever altered. True, this was their parent, whom many sons loved, and seeing the parent in this condition was very sad. However, a parent's growing old and becoming ill was somewhat expected. After their parents' deaths, sons would continue on with their work and families. Their lives would go on much like before the illness, unlike the husband caregivers', and the sons knew this.

Yet the sons' pain, anguish, frustration, and anger were ever present. Many sons lived with an overwhelming feeling of guilt that they had not done enough. As one son said, "I did not live up to my model of what a good son should be."

Nevertheless, sons, unlike the husband caregivers, were able to set boundaries and time limits on the caregiving. Often, when a parent reached the stage beyond which the son felt he was no longer able to provide the care, he looked for other options. Most often this option was a nursing home placement. Sons much sooner than husbands were willing to consider nursing home placement as a very real possibility.

Sons, on the whole, were more critical and demanding of services for their family members and themselves. They were more politically sophisticated and more active in patient and program advocacy, and their expectations were higher, a key intergenerational difference.

Sons more than husbands, however, came away with a feeling of satisfaction from their caregiving experience. Their parents' illness gave them an opportunity to "pay them back" for the years of love, care, and attention they had received, an opportunity that many sons believed they might never otherwise have had.

Thus, in general the sons' caregiving experiences were more conflicted, more complex, and more diverse than the husbands'. Husbands and their motivations for caregiving were more straightforward. As one husband caregiver insightfully summarized, "It all boils down to the two V's, vows and values." Such differences illustrate how much more needs to be understood about male caregivers.

Racial and Social Class Differences

Race and social class were not the predominant focus of this study. However, from the narratives some observations became apparent. Eighteen percent of the sample was African-American. Twenty-eight percent of the sample had incomes under $20,000 a year and 16 percent of the sample had incomes under $10,000.

For the most part, the caregiving experience of the husbands and sons were very similar across race and social class, as indicated throughout this book. The common themes and caregiving typologies of each group did not vary by race and social class. Other studies have also noted similarities in the ways African-American and white caregivers adapt to their caregiving role (Hinrichsen and Ramirez, 1992). But there were three key differences involving race and social class in this study.

Those male caregivers whose incomes were below $20,000 experienced more hardship in providing the care that their family members needed. A higher percentage of African-American caregivers than white caregivers in this sample fell into this category. Most services, such as respite care, were fee-for-service, and the caregivers in this income bracket could not afford them. A few of the caregivers could not afford the medications or medical care that might have helped their relatives with their multiple health care problems. For these men, dealing with their relatives' dementia was one more survival problem they needed to endure. As one African-American husband said, "I had a nice savings when I retired. Now I just have to get away from these doctor bills. I didn't owe one dime to nobody before this disease. And now I might have to sell this house. I built it myself."

A second difference was that the African-American men in the sample had more assistance from friends and neighbors in their caregiving than the white men in the sample, a finding supported by other research (Johnson and Barer, 1990). Friends and especially neighbors were an important source of emotional and hands-on support for this group of male caregivers. Both African-American sons and husbands remarked "how blessed" they were to have such friends, who often played the role of family, or "fictive kin." As a consequence, they were for the most part less socially isolated than the white men in the sample.

The third difference between the African-American and white male caregivers involved religion. Religion was a source of comfort and support for many white and African-American men in the study. Yet it had different meanings for the two groups, and it was practiced differently, as is also noted by other researchers (Levin, Taylor, and Chatters, 1994; Lincoln and Mamiya, 1990).

For the African-American men, their spirituality provided guidance for the difficult day-to-day decisions they needed to make in the caregiving. In times of utter despair, they would turn to God and look for some sort of a sign and direction about what to do next, how to handle the new challenge with which they were confronted. Their spirituality was an integral part of their daily lives. Quite often they were active members of their church, and the church's influence went beyond religion, extending into multiple areas of their lives: social, civic, political, and educational. For the African-American male caregivers, their religion was a combination of organized and nonorganized religious practice in spiritual and secular domains.

A number of the white men in the sample also found solace in their religion, but it was different. Their religious beliefs were not as all-encompassing in their everyday lives, and their religious activities focused more on organized religion. They attended church services regularly, and many participated in Communion. They found comfort sitting in silence in an empty church and thinking or talking to their clergy. Their religious life was more confined, and one of the consequences was that they participated in spiritual life differently. Yet the results were the same. Their religion was a source of great emotional support for them, too.

Thus, although the similarities among male caregivers that cut across race and social class lines were great, there were also some racial and social class differences.

Questions: Where Do We Go from Here?

Since so little research has been done on male caregivers, there are many questions that still need to be asked and answered as we delve into their world. This study begins the process. Some questions with which we are left are the following:

- Do the caregiving orientations used by husbands and sons change over time?
- What impact do the stages of dementia have on these caregiver orientations? The impact of the disease on the husband and son typologies needs to be further clarified.
- What motivates certain sons in a family to assume the responsibility for caring for a parent with dementia while other siblings seem unmotivated? Past relationships with the parent and geographic proximity do not seem to have the impact that one would expect.
- What role does religious affiliation have on caregiving?
- Do religions that have more of a salvation approach versus a social responsibility approach influence their adherents differently in providing motivation to assume the caregiving role for an ill family member?
- What is the impact of race and social class on the long-term caregiving experience?
- Do friends and neighbors continue to be a major source of support for African-American male caregivers as their ill relative moves into the latter stage of dementia? Or do the friends and

neighbors fade away, as is reported by most caregivers? Longitudinal analyses need to be done.

- What impact will the cuts in Social Security and Medicare have on the male caregivers in all areas of the economic spectrum? It is assumed that men are better off economically in our society, but what about men caring for severely impaired wives and parents? What impact does this care have on their financial security?

- How can service-delivery systems with fewer dollars for health and social services effectively and efficiently meet the changing needs of male caregivers?

- What new services can be developed to address the various needs of husbands and sons, given these stipulations?

- What about the other male caregivers whom this study does not address, male friends and neighbors, nephews and other male relatives, and long-distance caregivers? What is the extent of their involvement?

- Do the particular issues and concerns of sons trying to provide care to an ill parent hundreds of miles away also need to be considered in planning a comprehensive service-delivery system?

Finally, a cautionary word about the possibility of elder abuse by male caregivers must be mentioned. Although many men in the study were coping with the strain of caregiving, for others the demands of caregiving may have exceeded their coping skills. This fact can set the stage for the possibility of elder abuse. The question must be asked, How often does elder abuse occur among male caregivers? And are there certain types of male caregivers that are at higher risk for being abusers than others?

It is estimated that 1.5 million individuals are victims of elder abuse and neglect every year (Ashley and Fulmer, 1988). There was a 94 percent increase in the reported cases of elder abuse from 1986 to 1991, and most often the abusers were adult children or spouses (Tatara, 1993). This sample of male caregivers and their family members with dementia does have characteristics that have been identified as putting a family member at risk for the possibility of abuse. Factors that have been identified as contributing to an adult's increased vulnerability for abuse or neglect are advanced age—the older the adult, the more likely she or he will be a victim of abuse or neglect; cognitive and functional impairments; and sharing a household with the caregiver (Tatara, 1993; Godkin, Wolf, and Pillemer, 1995; Steinmetz, 1983). Caregiver characteristics identified as putting an individual at risk for becoming an abuser relevant to this sample are social isolation and lack of social supports; external stress due to financial and/or chronic health care problems; sudden and unexpected dependency; excessive stress; and unresolved family conflicts between older adult and caregiver (Hudson and Johnson, 1986; Godkin, Wolf, and Pillemer, 1995). In addition, Godkin, Wolf, and Pillemer (1995) in their small control group study did find that violence against the elderly is more likely to occur if men are caregivers, although because of sample size, the generalizability of this study is limited. There is no doubt that future research with male caregivers needs to explore these issues, too.

So much more needs to be known about men in their role of providers of care to relatives with dementia. We are just beginning to scrutinize and ask questions.

Our Final Reflections

Overhearing a chance conversation in an elevator was the spark that ignited this research on men caring for a relative with dementia. Four major questions evolved that guided the study: What is it like for a man to take on a major caregiving role? How does he adapt to and cope with his new functions? What are his motivations for taking on this role? And what meaning, if any, does he derive from it? This study moves us a little closer to answering these questions.

Each man in this study in his own way attempted to answer these questions and to add his own insights to what it is like for him, a husband or a son, to care for his wife or parent with dementia. The voices were many, and the situations and experiences varied.

There was the 43-year-old truck driver trying to help his wife maintain some control over life as she struggled with the ramifications of being diagnosed with early onset dementia. There was the 91-year-old physician who was "running out of steam" as he was dealing with his anger and frustration over what was now happening to his 89-year-old wife. There was the anguish of the 46-year-old business executive who "wanted to hold his father's hand" and be with him as he went through the end stage of his illness, but was prevented from doing so by his other obligations. And there was the 32-year-old son and his two sisters who had sacrificed 11 years of their lives to provide hands-on care to their mother in his home. Four men, four stories; sixty men, sixty stories—all very different, yet at the same time very similar.

What is it like for a man to take on a major caregiving role? It is different for a husband than a son, but a general picture starts to take shape. It is a complex image, with various levels of shading and intensity. The outline of this reflection is made up of an unwavering sense of commitment that holds the image together. Yet there is still a sense of the picture being out of control. At the center of this picture, a man demonstrates a wide range of emotions, from pain and anger to love and compassion. He struggles to express these feelings and deal with them. He learns new feminine roles, some of which come easily and others with much difficulty. He copes often with loss, role reversal, and social isolation, sometimes aided in his endeavors by his wife, children, siblings, and/or friends, but most often alone. He anchors himself by taking charge of his situation, by using a problem-solving approach, and often by finding solace in his religion. And out of this toil often comes a sense of satisfaction and a sense of personal growth, but a sense of utter despair may also come.

How does he cope and adapt? He does this by orienting his caregiving around a central motif that guides his life and gives him a sense of direction and meaning. It could be an orientation around a sense of duty, a deep commitment of love, a shared endeavor, or a work or strategic planning focus. He copes by adapting to his new role by whatever orientation works best for him. How does he find it? From his life experiences and knowledge of his own personal strengths, he usually finds it intuitively, although at times his accomplishments often surprise even himself.

What are his motivations? His major motivation is a deep sense of responsibility and obligation. It may be a "promise made years ago"; for some it is a "paying back for past caring"; for others "it is just what you do." His impetus for caregiving comes also out of love, devotion, loyalty, guilt, and acceptance of his responsibility as a birthright.

What meaning does he derive from the caregiving experience?

It provides him with a sense of purpose, a sense of usefulness—a raison d'être. It is a challenge placed before him to see how strong and how worthy he is. It is an opportunity to pay back a devoted parent or wife for years of care and devotion. But for some it can be a painful, tormenting, meaningless experience that "feels like you are standing on the rim of a big dark bottomless abyss and you're fighting from being sucked in."

We gained these insights about the male caregiving experience and so much more from these 60 men. Their reflections are scattered throughout the book. From their combined experiences, they could answer in one voice the single question that some men felt they were always being challenged with—"As a man, what do you know about caregiving?" These 60 men could answer, "Enough to know the pain, the despair, the anguish, the hardships, the satisfactions, and the hopes."

Appendix A
Interview Guides for Husband and Son Caregivers

Interview Guide for Husband Caregivers
Presented below are the topics divided into categories that were covered in the interviews with the 30 husbands. With the exception of the first topic, the others were not discussed in any particular sequence. The exact wording of these questions changed with the context of each interview.

Role as Caregiver
1. I've found the best way to get started is for you to tell me a little bit about your wife's situation and your involvement. Start from wherever makes sense to you.
2. What are your wife's diagnosis and symptoms? What are her level of impairment and the duration of her illness?
3. How would you define your caregiving role? How has it changed over time?
4. What has been the most difficult part of the experience for you?
5. Have you had any sense of satisfaction or accomplishment in this role?
6. What are some of the losses and disappointments that you have experienced in this process of caring for your wife?
7. What tasks have you taken on? What has been the most difficult task for you?
8. Have you had to learn new roles? How did you learn them?
9. What impact has your wife's dementia had on your life style and life plans?
10. How has your life changed?

Stress and Coping

11. What are some of the stresses you have experienced in caring for your wife? Have they changed over time?
12. What has helped you cope with some of the difficult situations?
13. Is there someone you turn to for help and support? Who is it and what does he/she do for you?
14. How has this illness had an impact on you financially?
15. What types of services have you used? Have they been helpful? Why or why not?
16. What have been the most helpful and least helpful services?
17. What suggestions do you have for new services for husbands caring for a wife with dementia?

Marital and Family Relationships

18. Tell me how this illness and your taking on this caregiving role has affected your relationship with your wife.
19. Has it affected your feelings of closeness and intimacy?
20. Tell me about your relationships with your children (past and present). How has impact of the disease changed these relationships?
21. What roles have your children played in helping you care for your wife?
22. What are your expectations of your children?
23. Do they understand the disease and accept the changes it has had on their mother? Explain more.
24. What have been the roles of other family members?

Meaning and Motivation

25. What made you decide to take on the day-to-day care of your wife?
26. Why do it?
27. What does the experience of caregiving mean to you? Have you made any sense out of it?
28. Has a sense of purpose developed? Explain.
29. Has it been a personal growth experience? Explain.

Interview Guide for Son Caregivers

Presented below are the topics divided into categories that were covered in the interviews with the 30 sons. The topics were not discussed in any particular sequence, and the exact wording of the questions changed with the context of each interview.

Role as Caregiver

1. I've found the best way to get started is for you to tell me a little about your parent's situation and your involvement. Start from wherever makes sense to you.
2. What are your parent's diagnosis and symptoms? What is the level of impairment and the duration of the illness?
3. How would you define your caregiving role? How has it changed over time?
4. What do you do for your parent; what tasks do you perform? How have these changed over time?
5. Have you had to learn new roles? What are they and how have you learned from them?
6. What has been the most difficult part of this experience for you?
7. What are some of the disappointments and losses you have experienced in the process of caring for your parent?
8. Have you had any sense of satisfaction or accomplishment in caring for your parent?
9. How has the caregiving affected your life style?
10. How has it affected your work?

Stress and Coping

11. What are some of the stresses you have experienced in caring for your parent? Have they changed over time?
12. What has helped you cope with some of the difficult situations?
13. Is there someone you turn to for help and support? Who is it and what does he/she do for you?
14. How has this illness had an impact on you and your parent financially?
15. What types of services have you used? Have they been helpful? Why or why not?
16. Tell me about the most helpful and least helpful services.

17. What suggestions do you have for new services for sons caring for a parent with dementia?

Family Relationships
18. Tell me about your relationship with your ill parent and well parent (if relevant) and how this illness has impacted it.
19. Tell me about the role(s) your siblings have played in caring for your parent (if not an only child).
20. Where do your siblings live?
21. Where are you in the birth order?
22. Has this experience affected your relationships? How?
23. Tell me about your wife's role in caring for your parent (if married).
24. What is her relationship with your ill parent?
25. What impact has your parent's illness had on your marriage?
26. What has been your children's role (where relevant) in caring for their grandparent?
27. Do they understand the disease and its impact on their grandparent?
28. What has been the impact of your parent's illness on your family?

Meaning and Motivation
29. Why have you taken on this caregiving role? Why you rather than your siblings?
30. What does the experience of caregiving mean to you? Have you made any sense of it?
31. Has it been a personal growth experience? Explain.

Appendix B
Characteristics of Husband and Son Caregivers

Table 1 Characteristics of Husband Caregivers (n=30)

	n	percent
Age in Years		
Mean	72.6	
Range	41–91	
Age of Wife in Years		
Mean	71.3	
Range	43–88	
No. of Years Married		
Mean	44.3	
Range	13–69	
Race		
White	24	80
African-American	6	20
*Level of Education**		
Less than high school	2	7
High school	11	38
College	16	55
Occupation		
Blue collar	12	40
Sales/Middle management	3	10
Professional/Business exec.	15	50
Employment Status		
Working	4	13
Retired[†]	26	87
Household Income		
Under $10,000	8	27
$11,000–$20,000	7	23
$21,000–$30,000	6	20
$31,000–$40,000	1	3
Over $40,000	8	27

Religion
Catholic	9	30
Jewish	2	7
Protestant	19	63

Living Arrangement
Lives alone with wife	21	72
Lives with wife and children	6	21
Lives separately	2	7

No. of years wife has had dementia
Less than 1 year	7	23
1–4 years	7	24
5 years or more	16	53
Mean	5.6	
Range	0.25–15	

Stage of dementia of wife[††]
Early	12	40
Middle	8	27
Late	10	33

Children in town
Yes	18	60
No	9	30
No children	3	10

Alzheimer's Disease Service Utilization[§]
Information and referral call	10	33
Educational literature	14	47
Educational programs	10	33
Support groups (attended more than 2)	18	60
Respite care	14	47
Day care	3	10
Nursing home	3	10
Financial/legal planning	6	20
Other	9	30

---

*n will vary due to missing data.
[†]No respondent retired to take care of his wife.
[††]Based on husbands' descriptions.
[§]Some respondents chose more than one.

Table 2 Characteristics of Son Caregivers (n=30)

	n	percent
Age in Years		
Mean	50	
Range	32–71	
Marital Status		
Married	18	60
Not married	12	40
Race		
White	25	83
African–American	5	17
Level of Education		
High school grad.	8	27
College	16	53
Advanced degree	6	20
Employment Status		
Working	23	77
Retired*	7	23
Occupation		
Blue collar	8	27
Sales/Middle management	6	20
Professional	8	27
Entrepreneur/Business exec.	8	27
Income		
Under $10,000	2	7
$11,000–$20,000	0	0
$21,000–$40,000	9	30
$41,000–$60,000	7	23
Over $60,000	12	40
Religion		
Catholic	17	57
Jewish	3	10
Protestant	8	27
No affiliation	2	6
Siblings in family		
Son only child	7	23
Has sisters	8	27
Has brothers	6	20
Has sisters and brothers	9	30
Geographic location of siblings		
Son only child in town	15	50
Sister(s) in town	6	20
Brothers(s) in town	2	7
Both in town	7	23

Birth Order		
Only	7	23
Oldest	5	17
Middle	9	30
Youngest	9	30
Sex of Parent		
Male	10	33
Female	20	67
Age of Parent in Years		
Mean	77	
Range	63–96	
Marital status of parent		
Married	13	43
Widowed/divorced	17	57
No. of years parent has had dementia		
Less than 1	5	16
1-4 years	17	57
5 years or more	8	27
Mean	3.5	
Range	5–11	
Parent's stage of dementia[†]		
Early	11	36
Middle	8	27
Late	5	17
Deceased	6	20
Living arrangements of parent		
Living alone	2	7
Living with spouse	6	20
With son	7	23
Other relatives' home	2	7
Nursing home	7	23
Deceased	6	20
Alzheimer's Disease Service Utilization[††]		
Information and referral call	23	76
Educational literature	21	70
Educational programs	10	33
Support groups (attended more than 2)	7	23
Respite care	7	23
Day care	7	23
Nursing home	8	26
Financial/legal planning	8	26
Other	5	16

*One respondent retired to take care of mother.
[†]Based on husbands' descriptions.
[††]Some respondents chose more than one.

Appendix C
Early Stage Programs

Chapter 4 discusses a specific type of early stage program that some of the husband caregivers found extremely helpful. This type of specialized support program includes the person with the illness as well as the caregiver. As people are being diagnosed earlier and informed of their diagnosis, more Alzheimer's Association chapters and other organizations are starting to provide specialized services for the person with the illness.

The following information is supplied as a guide to professionals who are interested in developing this type of program. Professionals are encouraged to contact Alzheimer's Association chapters and other social service organizations that have developed programs for diagnosed individuals to get complete information about the skills and tools necessary to develop this service. The sample information presented here was developed by the Alzheimer's Association–Cleveland Area Chapter, 12200 Fairhill Road, Cleveland, OH 44120, telephone: (216) 721–8457.

Something for You (Early Stage Program)

Something for You is an eight-week educational series for persons with early stage memory loss and their families. Topics include current research, tips on memory and how memory works, enlisting support, and common decisions individuals and their families face, such as driving, living arrangements, and legal and financial issues. Presenters include family members, physicians, researchers, and others. The program is facilitated by three professionals from the fields of social work or nursing who specialize in geriatrics, as well as one family co-leader. The meetings are two hours long, held at the same time during eight consecutive weeks. The series is offered twice a year. There is no charge for this series, but families must meet with a staff member before registration.

Something for You is a support and education series for

- persons with a diagnosis of irreversible memory loss.
- persons in the early stages and their family members and friends.
- persons who understand that they have a diagnosis of irreversible memory loss. They do not have to agree with the diagnosis.
- persons willing and able to express their questions and concerns.
- persons willing to make an eight-week commitment.

Key Screening Points

Diagnosis
- Diagnosis testing must be completed and all treatable causes ruled out prior to admission to the group.
- The diagnosis "Alzheimer's disease" does not have to be spelled out in the results of this testing. Persons who have related disorders are appropriate if these disorders are irreversible and progressive in nature. Dementia from a head injury, for example, would not usually be appropriate unless this injury had triggered another illness such as Alzheimer's disease. Very unique situations, such as a person in his/her thirties or someone with a related illness resulting in highly unusual symptoms or progression would not be a good candidate for this group.
- The person with memory loss does not have to accept that he/she has Alzheimer's disease but must acknowledge some difficulty with memory.

Communication Skills
- The person with memory loss may have difficulty finding the right word, but he/she must be able to express thoughts even if mostly in short phrases.
- He/she must have an interest in following what is being talked about and be able to comprehend, in a general sense, the meaning of what is being said.
- Sometimes a person's high social skills and sense of humor can more than compensate for limited verbal skills.
- The individual does not have to have a strong desire to talk

about his/her feelings. He/she must, however, be accepting of being in a group situation even if it will be mainly as an observer.

Attention Span

- The individual must be comfortable sitting through a two-hour session with one fifteen-minute break.
- This series utilizes breakout sessions in which diagnosed persons and family members meet in separate rooms. The person must be able to tolerate this separation.

Interest Level

- The individual does not have to have a high interest in attending the series. However, if he/she clearly has no interest in learning more about memory loss or meeting others in a similar situation, it is probably best not to enroll at this time.
- He/she must understand that this is an eight-week series and the importance of attending all eight sessions.

Alzheimer Association Chapters with Early Stage/Early Onset Support Programs

California

Marin County	(415) 472–4340
Orange County	(714) 283–1111
San Diego	(619) 537–5040
San Francisco	(415) 962–8111

Colorado

Rocky Mountain	(303) 813–1669

Florida

Orlando	(407) 422–9595

Hawaii

Honolulu	(808) 591–2771

Illinois

Chicago	(708) 933–2413

Massachusetts
Eastern   (617) 494–5150
Western   (413) 527–0111

Maryland
Baltimore/Central   (410) 561–9099

Washington, DC   (301) 652–6446

Michigan
Detroit   (810) 557–8277
South Central   (313) 741–8200

Minnesota
Minneapolis   (612) 888–7653

North Carolina
S. Piedmont   (704) 532–7392

Missouri
St. Louis   (314) 432–3422

New York
New York City   (212) 983–0700
Rochester   (716) 442–3820
Western New York   (716) 831–7084

Ohio
Cleveland   (216) 721–8457

Pennsylvania
Philadelphia   (215) 568–6430

Texas
Tarrant County   (817) 336–4949

Virginia
Northern   (703) 207–7044
Hampton Roads   (804) 459–2405

Appendix D
Computer Support Networks

Chapters 4 and 7 refer to computer support networks for Alzheimer's caregivers. Use of the computer, for some male caregivers, has proven to be a convenient and palatable method of receiving support and gathering information. The Alzheimer's Disease Support Center (ADSC) now can be accessed through the World Wide Web (WWW) on the Internet. The ADSC was developed by the Alzheimer Center of the University Hospitals of Cleveland/Case Western Reserve University and the Alzheimer's Association-Cleveland Area Chapter. The following are directions for how to get to the ADSC Web site:

To access the ADSC on the Cleveland Free-Net via the WWW,
> type: http://www.cwru.edu/orgs/adsc/intro.html
> click on: Cleveland Area Information and Events
> click on: The Alzheimer's Disease Support Center on the Cleveland Free-Net
> click on: Freenet-in-a.cwru.edu OR freenet-in-b.cwru.edu
You will then see the city motif . . . type 2 (to enter as a visitor) and then pick 1 to apply for an account on the Cleveland Free-Net OR 2 to explore the system. Once into the system type: Go Alz

The following shows how the Alzheimer's Disease Support Center is organized and the menu selections available:

Alzheimer's Disease Support Center
1. About the Support Center
2. Alzheimer's Disease Q & A
3. Alzheimer's Disease Information Rack
4. Alzheimer's Disease Bulletin Board

5. Alzheimer's Disease Caregiver Forum
6. The Professionals Forum
7. Alzheimer's Disease International Forum

Demographic Profile of Known DS Computer Support Network on the Cleveland Free-Net (as of January, 1996)

Age (n=138)
Range	10–84
Mean	51.4

Gender (n=189)
Female	134 (71%)
Male	55 (29%)

Race (n=189)
White	156 (83%)
African-American	33 (17%)

Relationship to Diagnosed (n=168)
Children and children-in-law	101 (60%)
Spouses	46 (27%)
Other (grandchildren, nieces, nephews, siblings, neighbors, etc.)	33 (17%)

Residence of Person with Dementia (n=138)
Home	72 (52%)
Nursing home	23 (17%)
Deceased	16 (12%)
With other family	15 (11%)
Alone	12 (9%)

Appendix E
Hiring In-Home Help

Both husbands and sons said they wanted more how-to information about securing in-home help for the person with dementia. The following are excerpts from two sources of information that represent the type of handouts/instruction for which these men said they were looking. They are meant to serve as an example of the type of specific how-to information that should be developed for this caregiving population.

The first selection is from the booklet "Caring for an Alzheimer's Disease Patient at Home: A Partnership Among the Family Caregiver, the Agency, and the Home Health Aide," by Emma Shulman, CSW, MP, and Gertrude Sternberg, MA, Aging & Dementia Research Center, New York University Medical Center, New York, New York; Sponsored by Jensen Pharmaceutic and distributed by the New York City chapter of the Alzheimer's Association. Reprinted by permission. The second excerpt is from a handout distributed by the Alzheimer's Association–Cleveland Area Chapter, developed by Margaret Kuechle, LISW. Reprinted by permission.

Caring for an Alzheimer's Disease Patient at Home
A Partnership Among the Family Caregiver, the Agency, and the Home Health Aide

Selecting the agency: Once you have decided to hire an aide, you need to determine how you will go about it. You may have heard from a friend, for example, of a very good aide who took care of a heart patient who has just died. You meet the aide, decide what your requirements are, and make "satisfactory" arrangements. On her first day of work, she phones you because her little girl is sick and she can't come in.

Naturally, that is the day both the patient and you have been up all night and the patient is tired and acting up. You have a crisis on your hands.

Unfortunately, this is a typical example of what can happen when a caregiver hires an aide directly. If emergencies or problems with the aide occur, you have nowhere to turn for help. Moreover, you must assume the burden of handling all the required taxes and insurance coverages.

We strongly recommend that you find an aide through an agency. By taking this path, you are really hiring the agency not the aide. You pay the agency and the agency pays the aide. The agency trains and supervises the aide, provides back-up in an emergency, pays all taxes (social security, withholding, unemployment, etc.), carries liability insurance for the aide, and sends you someone trained and experienced in caring for Alzheimer's patients.

There are a number of things you need to remember as you select an agency:

- If you have to sign an agreement or a contract, read the fine print carefully before signing. Ask questions.
- Sometimes, an agency may tell you that its aides are vendors—that they pay their own taxes and their own insurance. If you choose to use such an agency, make sure that you protect yourself by carrying workman's compensation. In addition, have the aide sign an agreement that he or she will pay all necessary federal, state, and city taxes and hope the tax department will accept this agreement.
- If an aide does not want you to pay Social Security or unemployment insurance, kindly but firmly insist on doing so. You could be held liable for those unpaid taxes.
- Before hiring an agency and an aide, check your health insurance policy. Most insurance, including Medicare, does *not* cover custodial care, which is the kind of care a home health aide gives. This care also may be called "nonmedical care."

Use this list of questions to help you interview an agency.

- How long has agency been in business?

- Does agency serve a large number of Alzheimer's patients?
- What is agency fee?
- What services are included in fee?
- What other services does agency offer and at what charge?
- How does agency handle payment and billing?
- Is there a minimum time and charge, e.g., 20 hours per week?
- Are aides covered by accident insurance and for how much?
- Does fee include assessment by a registered nurse?
- When is assessment made?
- Does fee include supervision by a registered nurse?
- How often does supervisor make home visits?
- Does supervisor call in advance to make appointment with caregiver?
- How much Alzheimer's disease training has aide had?
- Is a care plan made? When?
- What is rate if aide works overtime?
- What is the sleep-in rate?
- What holidays does aide get paid for and at what rate?
- Does agency provide back-up help in an emergency? How quickly?
- How much notice does agency give if aide is planning on leaving or going on vacation?
- Can agency provide references: For the agency? For the caregiver?

Hiring In-Home Help

The following material was prepared by the Alzheimer's Association–Cleveland Area Chapter. It was prepared for a caregiver's workshop held in October 1986. The material is designed to help a family member think through some of the issues involved when deciding to hire in-home help on his/her own. It is not intended to be comprehensive but is presented as an example of the type of information both husbands and sons said they wanted to have when confronted with these decisions.

Determining What Help Is Needed

At some point it has become clear that some routines of daily living are no longer being accomplished, or at least are done only with great difficulty. To determine what help is needed, you may want to list necessary routines and ask yourself what you can do alone, what your family is able and willing to do, and what is not being done. From this you can develop a job description for your worker.

Setting up a Job Description/Contract

The purpose of a job description or contract is to clarify the duties and responsibilities of both parties. Having a formalized agreement is essential if there is a dispute about salary, hours of work, tasks, etc. A contract/job description can always be revised or updated as needed. The more specific you can be in a contract, the less chance there is for confusion or disagreement. If the job involves technical skills such as lifting into the bath tub or giving medications, the worker should be trained and experienced [and licensed] in those skills.

Included here is a sample contract and a blank contract form. You will need to individualize your own contract to meet your and your worker's needs, so you may wish to add other items or leave out some that are listed.

Advertising

How Do You Go about Securing a Worker?

Probably the best way is a recommendation from a family member, friend, or someone you trust. Let them know you are looking. Your church or synagogue, or an organization you belong to, the Mayor's Office for Senior Citizens, or community agencies may be important resources. You may want to check the "Situations Wanted" section of the classified ads of your newspapers.

If none of these methods proves fruitful, then you can try advertising in the "Help Wanted" classified sections of the community newspapers, college newspapers, or organizations' newsletters. At a minimum, your ad should include hours needed, a brief description of duties, telephone numbers, and time to call. You could also mention preferences such as non-smoker or male/female, and wage offered.

Examples:
1). Grocery shopping, light housekeeping. 6 hrs. every Friday. Non-smoker. 555-5555 after 5 P.M.
2). Female needed part-time. Personal care, household chores. Flexible hours. 555-5555 between 9 A.M. and noon.

Sample Contract

Employment Contract Between

Employer: _Kriss Kross_

and Employee: _Lee Jones_

Salary: _$6.00_ per hour   Fringe benefits: _Bus fare, lunch provided_

Terms of Payment: When: _Every Friday_   How: _Check_

Hours of Work: From: _10 A.M._ to: _3 P.M._ on _Mon., Wed., Fridays_

Changes in Scheduled Hours Are Negotiable

Employee's Social Security Number: _111-11-1111_

Duties to be Performed

A. Household Tasks

Dust and vacuum once a week
Mop kitchen floor once a week
Change sheets once a week
Wash laundry once a week
Do food shopping once a week
Cook lunch on days present
Wash dishes after each meal

B. Personal Care Tasks

Assist with bath & shampoo
  once a week
Assist with physical exercises
Transport monthly to doctor
  appts.
Provide some socializing,
  conversation

Nonacceptable Behavior

Smoking while at work
Evidence of intoxication

Using foul language
Coming to work late

Termination

Each party will give two weeks' notice before terminating this contract. Reasons for termination without notice: theft, failure to carry out duties, evidence of non-acceptable behavior, endangering employer's health or safety. For work which is unsatisfactory, the employee will be given two warnings. If work continues to be unsatisfactory, a termination date will be set.

Signed:

_____   _____
         Employer   Employee

Date:_____   Date:_____

Address:_____   Address:_____

Phone:_____   Phone:_____

Contract

Employment Contract Between

Employer: _____

and Employee: _____

Salary: _____ per hour Fringe benefits: _____

Terms of Payment: When: _____ How:_____

Hours of Work: From: _____ to: _____ on _____

Changes in Scheduled Hours Are Negotiable

Employee's Social Security Number: _____

Duties to be Performed

A. Household Tasks   *B. Personal Care Tasks*

1._____   1._____

2._____   2._____

3._____   3._____

4._____   4._____

5._____   5._____

Nonacceptable Behavior

1._____   3._____

2._____   4._____

Termination

Each party will give two weeks' notice before terminating this contract. Reasons for termination without notice: theft, failure to carry out duties, evidence of non-acceptable behavior, endangering employer's health or safety. For work which is unsatisfactory, the employee will be given two warnings. If work continues to be unsatisfactory, a termination date will be set.

Signed:

_____   _____
Employer   Employee

Date:_____   Date:_____

Address:_____   Address:_____

Phone:_____   Phone:_____

Interviewing

You do not need to interview every person who calls in response to your ad or other contacts. When applicants call, you should describe the job in some detail as well as your expectations and the general wage range you are offering. You may want to ask if they have done this kind of work before or why they are interested in this job.

For those whom you feel are appropriate for the job, set a specific appointment time for an interview. It is recommended that you invite a family member or friend to be present for the interview. This can be very helpful both for moral support and in sorting out the information you obtain during the interview.

For the interview: Have a sample contract ready for the applicant to read. Record name, address, and the telephone number of applicant. Below are some suggested interview questions. Make up your own list of questions that meet your particular need.

- Where have you worked before? What kinds of things did you do?
- Tell me something about your hobbies, interests.
- How do you feel about caring for an elderly or disabled person?
- Have you ever provided care for a person similar to what this job requires?
- How do you feel about cooking and eating what someone else wants?
- How do you handle persons who are angry or violent?
- Why are you choosing to do this kind of work?
- What makes you uncomfortable or angry?
- What is your attitude about smoking, drinking, or using drugs?
- Is there anything in the job description which you would not do?
- What commitment to staying on this job are you willing to make?
- Please give me two work-related and one personal reference.

Review your check list (which follows) before ending the interview. If the applicant is obviously unsuited, be noncommittal about future contact. Remind a suitable applicant that you will need to check references before making a decision. Never hire someone without checking references!

Take time after your interview to jot down your notes and impressions. This is an important decision and your own personal reaction is vital to a successful match. Discuss your impressions with a family member or friend.

Interview Check List

This check list is to be used during the interview of a prospective employee and completed immediately.

1. Was the person on time for the interview?
2. Did the applicant and I agree on the terms and conditions of the contract?
3. Do I need to modify my contract before employing this person? How?
4. Did I get at least two references that I can call to verify his/her ability to perform needed services?
5. Did I say when I would probably notify the applicant of his/her acceptance or nonacceptance?
6. Do I have the name and telephone number of the applicant?
7. Did I feel comfortable or at ease with the person?
8. Did I note any mannerisms that made me uncomfortable? (Dress, behavior?)

Questions to Ask References

1. How long have you known the applicant? Dates? In what relationship?
2. What was his/her position?
3. Can you tell me more about his/her responsibilities?
4. How did the person get along with you and senior adults?
5. What were your impressions of him/her as a worker?
6. Did he/she show initiative, or wait to be told what to do?
7. Was the person reliable/dependable?
8. What were the applicant's strengths? Weaknesses?
9. Did you find him/her trustworthy and honest?
10. Were you aware of any problems with drugs or alcohol?
11. Is he/she still working for you? If not, would you re-hire?

Describe the job situation and ask reference if the applicant would be a good match for the position.

Hiring

Once an applicant is offered the job and accepts, the contract should be signed before the worker starts. Each party should have a copy of the signed contract.

Financial and Legal Considerations

When you become an employer there are a number of obligations that are yours. If you pay $50.00 or more per quarter of the year to an employee, you are required by law to withhold for Social Security benefits and make quarterly payments to the IRS. [Author's note: Current limits are $1,000 per year. Consult the IRS for up-to-date information.] (Exception: If the person you are hiring reports to the IRS as self-employed and pays his/her own social security.)

Also be aware that accidents can happen to your employee and you need to have insurance coverage for such accidents.

Below is a check list covering a number of specifics:

1. Discuss with your homeowner insurance agent your liability coverage as it applies to someone in your employment.
2. You have drawn up a contract agreement detailing rate of pay, days and hours of employment. Also clarify fringe benefits— for example, bus fare.
3. Contact the IRS and get IRS forms and publications about current social security withholding requirements.
4. Set up a form for record of payments to employee (see below).
5. When you file your own 1040 tax return, determine if payments to your employee qualify as a medical deduction on your return.
6. Be aware of possible legal and financial pitfalls of paying cash instead of by check. Use receipt forms or other proof of payments to worker. (Generic receipt books are available where stationery supplies are sold.)
7. Keep a record of any serious problems you have with your worker, in case of dispute later.

Keeping Your Worker

Communication between employer and employee is important. People appreciate being told when doing a good job. It is also helpful to tell people about irritating factors. The small annoyances often cause problems when not discussed. A good work environment will generally bring the best performance from an employee. Open communication is a necessary component in providing a good work environment.

The following "tips" (suggestions/recommendations) should be considered in keeping communication open:

1.   Give praise for a job well done. People like to be appreciated.
2.   Be fair and kind.
3.   Respect your employee's privacy.
4.   Be sincere. Don't say something you don't mean—it might back-fire later.
5.   Be sure your employee understands what you expect. Give clear directions.
6.   When a worker does not know how to do a task requested, either you or a family member or friend should demonstrate what is desired. Have your worker demonstrate back to your satisfaction.
7.   Don't let small irritations build up until an angry confrontation occurs.
8.   Permit ample time for discussion to resolve problems.
9.   Treat your employee as you would like to be treated.

Giving Praise—Factors to Consider
Describe the situation or event you like and include your feelings. Examples:

•   "Thank you for putting non-skid strips in the bath tub. I feel so much safer." (Often "thank you" is all one needs to say.)
•   "I really appreciate the extra care you take in cleaning under the sofa, bed, and around the sink. Having a clean home is wonderful."
•   "Thank you very much for making the effort to be here on time."
•   "You certainly know how to give a nice manicure."

Giving Criticism—Factors to Consider
1.   Describe the situation or event you did not like. Include your feelings.

2.   Make a suggestion that would improve the situation next time.

3.   Many times it is better to give praise first and then follow with criticism.

Examples (Poor and Better):

> Poor—"It is not necessary to use ten rags to clean the kitchen floor and cupboards! Even though you wash the rags out, it annoys me to find rags pasted on all the counters—it looks so messy."

> Better—"You did a good job cleaning the kitchen floor and cupboards. But I'd like you to use fewer rags and hang them on the lines in the furnace room to dry after you've washed them out."

Use criticism as a tool to share information that will help do the job well:

1.   Give criticism as soon as possible after the problem occurs.

2.   Criticize only one incident at a time.

3.   Keep criticism brief and to the point.

4.   Criticize actions, not the person. (For example, "You are a terrible cook" criticizes the person; better to say "You cooked my eggs too long–I prefer softer eggs," which criticizes the action and suggests improvement.)

5.   Remember to forgive and forget.

Decision Tree: Do I Need Help in My Home?

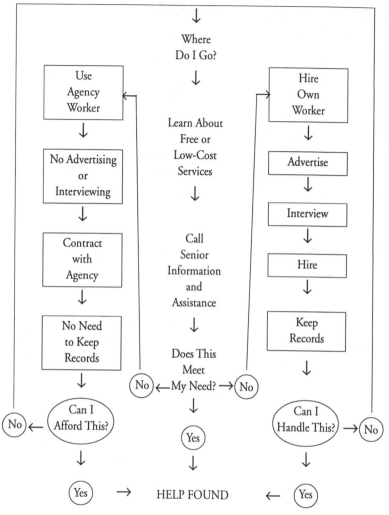

↓

Where
Do I Go?

↓

Use Agency Worker	Learn About Free or Low-Cost Services	Hire Own Worker
↓	↓	↓
No Advertising or Interviewing	Call Senior Information and Assistance	Advertise
↓	↓	↓
Contract with Agency		Interview
↓	↓	↓
No Need to Keep Records	Does This Meet My Need?	Hire

No ← My Need? → No

Can I Afford This? — Yes

No ←

Yes

↓ Yes

Can I Handle This? → No

Yes → HELP FOUND ← Yes

From: Cleveland Area Chapter Alzheimer's Association and Margaret Kuechle, LISW.

Appendix F
Evaluating Adult Day Care Services

The following is an example of the type of evaluation tool male caregivers requested to help them evaluate adult day care services. It is excerpted from the Alzheimer's Association–Cleveland Area Chapter's handout entitled "Adult Day Centers" by Joanne Frances Durante. Reprinted by permission.

Adult day centers provide socialization, stimulating activities, and a nutritious meal for persons who may need supervision or assistance in performing daily tasks. Adult day care also provides respite for caregivers. Adult day care can lift participants out of isolation and depression. Many families and adult day care workers notice that the functioning of adult day care participants with early Alzheimer's disease improves.

Adult day care centers run the gamut from small informal facilities in community centers or churches to large, professionally managed programs. Some centers have specialized adult day care programs for persons with Alzheimer's disease.

Here is a list of questions to help you determine if a specific adult day center can meet your needs:

- Is it convenient and accessible?
- Does it provide transportation?
- Are its service hours convenient for you?
- How much does it cost? Is financial assistance available?
- Are there hidden expenses such as craft supplies or outing fees?
- What is the policy on late arrival or late pick-up?
- What is the ratio of staff to participants? (The Ohio Association of Adult Day Care recommends a minimum ratio of 1:6.)

- What training does the staff have?
- Is there a warm and welcoming atmosphere?
- Are the staff and facility neat, clean and orderly?
- Are the meals nutritious and attractively prepared?
- Is there an initial assessment, including an evaluation of the person's health profile, social history, mental and social function, interests and needs?
- Is there a process for reviewing and updating the person's care plan?
- Does the center serve various levels of impairment?
- Is there a specialized program for persons with dementia? What makes this program special?
- Can the center accommodate special physical or medical requirements, such as:
  - special dietary needs
  - medication reminder
  - help with toileting
  - access and full participation for persons in wheelchairs?
- Is there a variety of planned recreational and social activities?
- Are there activities suitable to your person's interests and capabilities? For example:
  - an exercise program
  - music and dance
  - volunteer projects
  - creative arts
  - homemaker crafts
  - mental stimulation
  - indoor and outdoor gardening
  - cultural activities
  - joint activities with children
- Are there adequate space and furnishings for indoor and outdoor activities?
- How does the staff handle a person's unwillingness to actively participate?
- Are the participants potentially compatible with your family member's social history? (Some men are uncomfortable with a mostly female group; some people are intolerant of racial and ethnic differences. You need to be honest about this.)

- Are there specific behaviors or care needs which would compel withdrawal from the program? Since Alzheimer's disease is a progressive disorder, you need to find out not only how a facility handles existing care needs but also whether it can handle potential ones such as incontinence, agitation, or wandering.

Tips on Ensuring Day Center Success

- Don't wait until the person's social skills are seriously impaired; early involvement seems highly conducive to success.
- Introduce the day center experience in simple terms the person can understand and accept. For some, this means being direct about your own needs for time alone; others may find it helpful to emphasize the benefits of physical exercise or the social benefits of getting out and being with people; for others, emphasizing the opportunity to help others and stay busy are the keys.
- Share with the staff information on those activities your family member enjoys.
- Don't expect the person with dementia to remember or report on daily activities. If you are concerned about participation, talk to the program's social worker, director or family liaison person. How frequently a day center should be used is based on the need and on the degree of support/acceptance by the participant and family. Too few days may make acceptance difficult since continuity and a predictable routine are essential, but plunging into a five-day week may cause feelings of abandonment. Work with the staff to come up with a tentative schedule, and adjust it with time and experience as your needs change.
- Adjustment takes time. Be firm in your expectation that your family member will attend. Don't ask if he or she wants to go to the center today. Say, "Today's your day center (or 'club' or 'work') day." Suggest trying it for a month.
- Be on time and reliable about picking up and dropping off your family member. Reinforce with him or her the dependable predictability of this new routine.
- Share with the staff any changes in the person's medical or social situation as they occur.

Your support and acceptance of the day center experience may be the primary determinant of the person's success in this new environment. Your family member needs to know that his participation is beneficial for himself, you, and others. For the caring family, learning and accepting these facts will be the turning point in realizing positive benefits from the day center experience.

Appendix G
Alzheimer's Care in Residential Settings

The following is a sample of the type of information that male caregivers might find helpful in evaluating long-term care services. This information is provided only as an example of the type of instrument to which male caregivers, particularly sons, should be directed. The following is excerpted from the December 1992 edition of "Family Guide for Alzheimer's Care in Residential Settings," a booklet produced by the Alzheimer's Association, 919 North Michigan Avenue, Suite 100, Chicago, IL 60611-1676. Reprinted by permission.

Alzheimer's Care in Residential Settings Check List

I. Philosophy—What is "special" about Alzheimer's care? (yes/no)
1. Does the Alzheimer's care mission statement indicate benefits for you and your family member?
2. Are religious, cultural and unique advantages apparent for your family member?
3. Does the separated dementia unit or Alzheimer's care program offer special advantages for your family member?
4. Does the facility have licenses you consider necessary? (State licensure? Medicare certification? Medicaid certification? Private accreditations?)

II. Pre-admission—Selecting a facility
5. Is a specialized Alzheimer's/dementia care program available?
6. Is the facility location convenient for you?
7. Do you consider that the Alzheimer's care program admission requirements are acceptable?

8. Do other residents have functional capabilities similar to those of your family member?

9. Is assessment done by staff to determine individual special (Alzheimer's/dementia) care needs?

10. Is the program limited by discharge and/or transfer criteria?

11. Do you sense a caregiving partnership with facility staff?

12. Are resident rights addressed?

13. Is medical care and supervision sufficient?

14. Are behaviors accommodated without use of restraints?

15. Are fees and charges justified and competitive within your community?

16. Is Medicaid or other reimbursement available?

III. Admission—Entering the Facility

17. Do you feel support for your needs and concerns?

18. Are residents assisted by staff, volunteers and family?

19. Are advance directives (durable powers of attorney for health care and other determined instructions) discussed, documented and honored?

20. Is autopsy (for confirmation of diagnosis) discussed and family wishes honored?

IV. Care Planning and Implementation—Daily Living

21. Will you share in developing and reviewing an individualized care plan?

22. Is care planning done by an interdisciplinary care planning team?

23. Are care planning meetings held regularly and/or when needed to positively address care issues?

24. Is there a full daily schedule of therapeutic activities?

25. Are nutrition and eating needs of residents accommodated?

V. Change in Condition Issues—Disease Progression and Other Illness

26. Will diminished abilities result in transfer or discharge from the program?

27. Is late stage care and illness addressed?

VI. Staffing Patterns and Training—Staff Assignment and Alzheimer's Knowledge

28. Do you feel confident and comfortable with staff leadership?
29. Is Alzheimer's/dementia specific training available for all staff?
30. Does the number of staff appear adequate?
31. Are staff pleasant and encouraging to residents?
32. Is there competent monitoring of medical care?

VII. The Physical Environment—A Place for Alzheimer's Care

33. Is the environment safe and comfortable?
34. Does the size of the program offer benefits?
35. Is outdoor space available and used?
36. Is private space personalized and respected?
37. Is the environment calm and pleasurable?
38. Do safety measures meet the needs of your family member?

VIII. Success Indicators—Benefits of Alzheimer's Care

39. Do residents appear relaxed and content?
40. Are residents active and engaged in activities?
41. Is the atmosphere cheerful and homey?
42. Are residents clean and well groomed?
43. Do residents appear alert?
44. Are residents treated with dignity and respect?
45. Is restraint use absent or appropriate and closely monitored?
46. Are privacy needs and confidentiality respected?
47. Is there open communication among residents, families and staff?
48. Are research opportunities explained?
49. Is the Alzheimer's care program objectively evaluated?
50. Are all aspects of care supervised and evaluated?

Appendix H
A Sample Care Management Program

As noted in Chapter 7, caregiving sons expressed a desire for individualized professional advice in the care and management of their parents. The following information is supplied as a sample care management program that was instituted in the state of Ohio in 1993. It currently is provided at four Alzheimer's Association sites (Cincinnati, Cleveland, Columbus, and Youngstown). This program, called Getting Started, was partially funded by Grant #CSH00157-01-0 from the Health Resource and Services Administration, Department of Health and Human Services, and is administered by the Ohio Department of Aging. Professionals interested in receiving more information about Getting Started can contact the Ohio Department of Aging, 50 West Broad Street, Columbus, Ohio 43266-0501, (614) 644-7967 or the Cleveland Area Alzheimer's Association, 12200 Fairhill Road, Cleveland, Ohio 44120, (216) 721-8457.

Getting Started: A Resource and Planning Service to Strengthen Caregiving Families

Getting Started provides an opportunity for members of a caregiving family to come together for personalized assistance in:

- Identifying immediate needs
- Learning about community services and how best to use them
- Developing a plan of action.

Initial meetings with the Getting Started coordinator can be held at the Alzheimer's Association office, in the family home, or at another convenient location.

There is no charge for Getting Started.

Upon referral, the Getting Started coordinator (a social work professional with geriatric experience) arranges a meeting with the primary and secondary caregivers and any other interested family members as possible. Meetings range from one to two hours and focus on the specific issues and concerns of that caregiving family. Family strengths as well as problems are examined. The coordinator helps families learn how to prioritize their needs. Referrals are made to link families not only to the formal support network (day care, in-home respite, nursing homes, etc.) but also to the local informal or natural support network that is often ignored or underutilized (neighbors, church groups, social contacts, etc).

Family members, with the assistance of the coordinator, develop a concrete action plan with specific tasks and assignments. All family members present are asked to sign off on the action plan. Specific follow-up intervals are agreed upon with the coordinator, who follows up with a designated family member by phone.

Getting Started does not replace other existing programs in the community but acts as a bridge to these other services. Families find the personalized nature of the service and the written action plan a unique and helpful tool in coping with their caregiving duties.

GETTING STARTED
Sample Action Plan for Family Members/Friends of
Jane Doe
(Name of Person with Dementia)

I. Primary Issues and Concerns

Mrs. Doe, although recently diagnosed with Alzheimer's Disease, is very confused and there are concerns about her living alone. She is widowed and depends on her care from her son, John, who lives nearby, and a daughter, Judy, who lives a half-hour away. John has questions about the illness, legal matters, and available home care.

II. Our Family's Strengths

Family has been very close over the years. John works but has a flexible schedule. John and Judy are very protective of their mother. John, Judy and their spouses all were willing to meet together and are open about care options.

III. Short Term Goals

1. Get information on legal planning.
2. Discuss safety issues and plan how to shut off the kitchen stove.
3. Relieve caregiver stress through respite services.
4. Family education on Alzheimer's disease.

IV. Tasks Required to Meet Short Term Goals

Task	Who	When
1. Attend legal planning seminar to be held next month.	John	April 16
G.S. coordinator will send hand-outs on legal issues.	G.S. Coor.	March 25
2. Purchase stove switch and contact recommended installer.	Judy	Within next 2 weeks
3. Contact Council on Aging for Alzheimer's respite program. 1-800-555-5555	John	Within next 2 weeks
4. View family education video (provided by G.S. Coordinator) for guidance on communication and behavior management.	John, Judy	Within next month
5. Attend Spring caregiver workshop.	John, Judy	April 25

V. Others Who Might Be Able to Help

John's wife, June and their teenage daughter Julie.
Judy's husband, Jim, is willing to watch Mrs. Doe on Saturday mornings.
Mrs. Doe's neighbor, Mrs. Smith, has expressed a desire to help out. Judy will talk with her and see if she is willing to spend a few hours a month with Mrs. Doe for companionship.

VI. Follow-up (When? Where? How?)

The Getting Started Coordinator will follow up in one month by telephone to John.

Date	Signatures	Relationship to Patient
March 15	Judy Doe James	daughter
March 15	Jim James	son-in-law
March 15	John Doe	son
March 15	June Doe	daughter-in-law
March 15	Susan Williams	Getting Started Coordinator

References

Abel, E.K. (1991). *Who cares for the elderly: Public policy and experiences of adult daughters*. Philadelphia: Temple University Press.

Allen, S.M. (1994). Gender differences in spousal caregiving and unmet need for care. *Journal of Gerontology: Social Sciences, 49*(4), S187–S195.

Ashley, J., and Fulmer, T.T. (1988). No simple way to determine elder abuse. *Geriatric Nursing, 9*(5), 286–288.

Barer, B.M. (1994). Men and women aging differently. *International Journal of Aging and Human Development, 38*(1), 29–40.

Bem, S.L. (1976). Probing the promise of androgyny. In A.G. Kaplan and J.P. Bean (eds.), *Beyond sex role stereotypes: Readings toward a psychology of androgyny* (pp. 47–62). Boston: Little, Brown.

Bertaux, D. (1981). *Biography and society: The life history approach in the social sciences*. Newbury Park, CA: Sage Publications.

Boles, J., and Tatro, C. (1982). Androgyny. In K. Solomon & N.B. Levy (eds.), *Men in transition* (pp. 99–129). New York: Plenum Press.

Borden, W., and Berlin, S. (1990). Gender, coping, and psychological well-being in spouses of older adults with chronic dementia. *American Journal of Orthopsychiatry, 60*(4), 603–610.

Brody, E.M. (1990). *Women in the middle*. New York: Springer.

Brody, E.M., Hoffman, C., Klaben, M.H., and Schoonover, C.B. (1989). Caregiving daughters and their local siblings: Perceptions, strains, and interactions. *The Gerontologist, 29*(4), 529–538.

Brody, E.M., Klaben, M.H., Johnsen, P.T., Hoffman, C., and Schoonover, C.B. (1987). Work status and parental care: A comparison of four groups of women. *The Gerontologist, 27*, 201–208.

Cantor, M.H. (1983). Strain among caregivers: A study of experience in the United States. *The Gerontologist, 23*, 597–604.

The Commonwealth Fund. (1993). The untapped resource: Final report of the Americans over 55 at Work program. New York: The Commonwealth Fund.

Coverman, S., and Sheley, J. (1986). Change in men's housework and child-care time, 1965–1975. *Journal of Marriage and the Family, 48* (May), 413–422.

Doty, P. (1986). Family care of the elderly: The role of public policy. *Milbank Memorial Fund Quarterly, 64*, 34–75.

Dulac, G., and Kosberg, J.I. (1994). Elderly men in North America: Changes and challenges. Paper presented at the 43rd Annual Scientific Meeting of the Gerontological Society of America, Atlanta, Georgia.

Dwyer, J.W., and Coward, R.T. (1991). A multivariate comparison of the involvement of adult sons versus daughters in the care of impaired parents. *Journal of Gerontology, 46*(5), S258–S269.

Farran, C.J., Keane-Hagerty, E., Salloway, S., Kupferer, S., and Wilken, C.S. (1991).

Finding meaning: An alternative paradigm for Alzheimer's disease family caregivers. *The Gerontologist, 31*(4), 483–489.

Finley, N.J., Roberts, D., and Banahan, B.F. (1988). Motivators and inhibitors of attitudes of filial obligation toward aging parents. *The Gerontologist, 28*(1), 73–78.

Fitting, M., Rabins, P., Lucas, M.J., & Eastham, J. (1986). Caregivers of dementia patients: A comparison of husbands and wives. *The Gerontologist, 26*, 248–252.

Fontana, A., and Frey, J.H. (1994). Interviewing: The art of science. In N.K. Denzin and Y.S. Lincoln (eds.), *Handbook of qualitative research* (pp. 361–375). Newbury Park, CA: Sage Publications.

Frankel, V.E. (1963). *Man's search for meaning.* New York: Washington Square Press.

———. (1978). *The unheard cry for meaning.* New York: Washington Square Press.

George, L.K. (1984). The burden of caregiving: How much? What kinds? For what? *Advances in Research, 8*(2). Durham, NC: Duke University, Center for the Study of Aging and Human Development.

George, L.K., and Gwyther, L. (1986). Caregiver well-being: A multidimensional examination of family caregivers of demented adults. *The Gerontologist, 26*, 253–259.

Gihooly, M.L.M. (1984). The impact of caregiving on caregivers: Factors associated with the psychological well-being of people supporting a demented relative in the community. *British Journal of Medical Psychology, 57*, 35–44.

Gilligan, C. (1982). *In a different voice: Psychological theory and women's development.* Cambridge, MA: Harvard University Press.

Glaser, B., and Strauss, A. (1967). *The discovery of grounded theory.* Chicago: Aldine.

Godkin, M.A., Wolf, R.S., and Pillemer, K.A. (1995). A case comparison analysis of elder abuse and neglect. In J. Hendricks (ed.). *The ties of later life* (pp. 113–130). Amityville, NY: Baywood Publishing.

Haley, W.E., Clair, J.M., and Saulsberry, K. (1992). Family caregiver satisfaction with medical care of their demented relatives. *The Gerontologist, 32*(2), 219–226.

Harris, P.B. (1993). The misunderstood caregiver?: A qualitative study of the male caregiver of Alzheimer's disease victims. *The Gerontologist, 33*(4), 551–556.

———. (1995). Differences among husbands caring for their wives with Alzheimer's disease: Qualitative findings and counseling implications. *Journal of Clinical Geropsychology, 1*(2), 97–106.

Harrison, J. (1978). Warning: The male sex role may be dangerous to your health. *Social Issues, 34*, 65–86.

Himes, C.L. (1992). Future caregivers: Projected family structures of older persons. *Journal of Gerontology: Social Sciences, 47*(l), 517–526.

Hinrichsen, G.A., and Ramirez, M. (1992). Black and white dementia caregivers: A comparison of their adaptation, adjustment and service utilization. *The Gerontologist, 32*(3), 375–381.

Horowitz, A. (1985). Family caregiving to the frail elderly. *Annual Review of Gerontology and Geriatrics, 5*, 194–246.

———. (1992). Methodological issues in the study of gender within family caregiving relationships. In J.W. Dwyer and R.T. Coward (eds.), *Gender, families, and elder care* (pp. 132–150). Newbury Park, CA: Sage Publications.

Hudson, M.F., and Johnson, T.F. (1986). Elder neglect and abuse: A review of the literature. *Annual Review of Gerontology and Geriatrics, 6*, 81–134.

Johnson, C.L. (1983). Dyadic family relations and social support. *The Gerontologist, 23*, 377–383.

Johnson, C.L., and Barer, B.M. (1990). Families and networks among older inner city blacks. *The Gerontologist, 30*, 726–740.

Kaye, L.W., and Applegate, J.S. (1990a). *Men as caregivers to the elderly: Understanding and aiding unrecognized family support.* Lexington, MA: Lexington Books.

———. (1990b). Men as elder caregivers: Building a research agenda for the 1990's. *Journal of Aging Studies, 4*(3), 289–298.

———. (1994). Older men and the family caregiving orientation. In E.H. Thompson (ed.), *Older men's lives* (pp. 218–236). Newbury Park, CA: Sage Publications.

Levin, J.S., Taylor, R.J., and Chatters, L. (1994). Race and gender differences in religiosity among older adults: Findings from four national surveys. *Journal of Gerontology: Social Sciences, 49*(3), S137–S145.

Lee, G.R., Dwyer, J.W., and Coward, R.T. (1993). Gender differences in parent care: Demographic factors and same gender preferences. *Journal of Gerontology: Social Sciences, 48* (I), S9–SI6.

Lincoln, C.E., and Mamiya, L.H. (1990). *The black church in the African American experience.* Durham, NC: Duke University Press.

McFadden, S.H. (1994). Empathy and caregiving. Paper presented at the 43rd Annual Scientific Meeting of the Gerontological Society of America, Atlanta, Georgia.

Miller, B. (1987). Gender and control among spouses of the cognitively impaired: A research note. *The Gerontologist, 27,* 447–453.

———. (1990). Gender differences in spouse management of the caregiver role. In E.K. Abel and M.K. Nelson (eds.), *Circles of care: Work and identity in women's lives* (pp. 92–104). Albany: State University of New York Press.

Miller, B., and Cafasso, L. (1992). Gender differences in caregiving: Fact or artifact? *The Gerontologist, 32*(4), 498–507.

Montgomery, R. (1995). Molding interventions to the caregiver's mosaic. Paper presented at the Center for Practice Innovations Conference, Case Western Reserve University, Cleveland, Ohio.

Montgomery, R., and Kamo, Y. (1987). Differences between sons and daughters in parental caregiving. Paper presented at the 36th Annual Scientific Meeting of the Gerontological Society of America, Washington, DC.

Motenko, A.K. (1988). Respite care and pride in caregiving: The experience of six older men caring for their disabled wives. In S. Reinhatz and G. Rowles (eds.), *Qualitative gerontology* (pp. 104–126). New York: Springer.

Mui, A.C. (1995). Caring for frail elderly parents: A comparison of adult sons and daughters. *The Gerontologist, 35*(1), 86–93.

Oakley, A. (1981). Interviewing women: A contradiction in terms. In H. Roberts (eds.), *Doing feminist research* (pp. 30–61). London: Routledge and Kegan Paul.

O'Neil, J.M. (1982). Gender role conflict and strain in men's lives. In K. Solomon and N.B. Levy (eds.), *Men in transition* (pp. 5–44). New York: Plenum Press.

Osgood, N.J. (1985). *Suicide in the elderly.* Rockville, MA: Aspen System Corporation.

Pearlin, L.I., and Schooler, C.E. (1978). The structure of coping. *Journal of Health and Behavior, 19,* 2–21.

Pearlin, L.I., Mullan, J., Semple, J., and Skate, M. (1990). Caregiving and the stress process: An overview of concepts and their measures. *The Gerontologist, 30,* 583–594.

Ruddick, S. (1989). *Maternal thinking: Toward a politics of peace.* Boston: Beacon.

Schultz, R. (1990). Theoretical perspectives on caregiving. Concepts, variables, and methods. In D.E. Biegel and A. Blum (eds.), *Aging and caregiving: Theory research and policy* (pp. 27–52). Newbury Park, CA: Sage Publications.

Shanas, E. (1979). Social myth as an hypothesis: The case of family relations of old people. *The Gerontologist, 19,* 3–9.

Shanas, E., and Strieb, G.F. (1965). *Social structure and the family: Generational relations.* Englewood Cliffs, NJ: Prentice-Hall.

Scharlach, A., Lowe, B., and Schneider, E. (1991). *Elder care and the work force: Blueprint for action.* Lexington MA: Lexington Books.

Smyth, K.A., and Harris, P.B. (1993). Using telecomputing to provide information and support to caregivers of persons with dementia. *The Gerontologist, 33*(1), 123–127.

Solomon, K. (1982). The older man. In K. Solomon and N.B. Levy (eds.), *Men in transition* (pp. 205–240). New York: Plenum Press.

Steinmetz, S.K. (1983). Dependency, stress, and violence between middle-aged caregivers and their elderly parents. In J.L. Kosberg (ed.), *Abuse and maltreatment of the elderly.* Littleton, MA: John Wright PSG, Inc.

Stoller, E.P. (1983). Parental caregiving by adult children. *Journal of Marriage and the Family, 45*, 851–858.

———. (1990). Males as helpers: The role of sons, relatives, and friends. *The Gerontologist, 33*(2), 228–235.

———. (1992). Gender differences in the experiences of caregiving spouses. In J.W. Dwyer and R.T. Coward (eds.), *Gender, families, and elder care* (pp. 49–64). Newbury Park, CA: Sage Publications.

Stone, R., Cafferata, G., and Sangl, J. (1987). Caregivers of the frail elderly: A national profile. *The Gerontologist, 29*, 677–683.

Tatara, T. (1993). *Summaries of the statistical data on elder abuse in domestic settings for FY 1990 and FY 1991.* Washington, DC: National Aging Resource Center on Elder Abuse.

Tennstedt, S.L., McKinlay, J.B., and Sullivan, L.M. (1989). Informal care for frail elders: The role of secondary caregivers. *The Gerontologist, 29*(5), 677–683.

Toseland, R.W., and Rossiter, C.M. (1989). Group interventions to support family caregivers: A review and analysis. *The Gerontologist, 29*(4), 438–448.

U.S. Bureau of the Census. (1989). Projections of the population of the United States by age, sex, and race: 1988–2080. Current Population Reports, Series P.25, No. 1018. Washington, DC: U.S. Government Printing Office.

U.S. Senate Special Committee on Aging. (1987). Developments in Aging. Washington, DC: U.S. Government Printing Office.

Vinick, B.H. (1984). Elderly men as caretakers of wives. *Journal of Geriatric Psychiatry, 17*(1), 61–68.

Weinstein, G.W. (1993, October). Help wanted—the crisis of elder care, *Ms. Magazine*, 73–79.

Wright, L.K. (1991). The impact of Alzheimer's disease on the marital relationship. *The Gerontologist, 31*, 224–237.

Young, R.F., and Kahana, E. (1989). Specifying caregiver outcomes: Gender and relationship aspects of caregiver strain. *The Gerontologist, 29*, 660–666.

Zarit, J.M. (1982). Predictors of burden and stress for caregivers of senile dementia patients. Unpublished doctoral dissertation, Univeristy of Southern California, Los Angeles, California.

Zarit, S., Todd, P.A., and Zarit, J.M. (1986). Subjective burden of husbands and wives as caregivers: A longitudinal study. *The Gerontologist, 26*, 260–266.

Index

Abel, E.K., 1
Adult day care services, 47, 166, 205–208
Allen, S.M., 6, 7
Alzheimer's disease
  acceptance of, 23, 48, 56–57, 68, 69–70, 96–97, 114, 121–122, 125, 145
  early onset, 9, 53, 66
  legal/financial planning for, 122 126, 152, 162
  reaction to diagnosis, 21–22
  special care units, 209–211
  stages of, 17–18
Applegate, J.S., 1, 7
Ashley, J., 174

Banahan, B.F., 92
Barer, B.M., 2, 5, 172
Bem, S.L., 6
Berlin, S., 3
Bertaux, D., 9
Boles, J., 6
Borden, W., 3
Brody, E.M., 1, 7, 92

Cafasso, L., 2
Cafferata, G., 2, 3
Cantor, M.H., 1
Caregiving
  acceptance of, 23, 48, 141–142, 150, 170
  care management, 163–165, 213–215
  commitment to, 21, 38, 42–43, 46–47, 51–52, 54, 60, 87, 91, 126, 128–129, 133, 153
  duty, 46–53, 95–96
  emotional reactions to, 22–24, 26, 40, 44, 45, 54, 99–102, 111–112, 129–130, 133

hope, 32
loss, 25–26, 39–40, 41, 44, 103, 170
meaning of, 31–32, 47, 108–109
positive impact of, 31–32, 42, 108–109
racial differences in, 171–173
reaction to medical diagnosis, 21–22
social isolation of, 24, 45, 130, 133
social support for, See Social supports
stress and burden of, 8, 24, 29–30, 102, 131, 133
Chatters, L., 172
Children
  role of adult children, 20, 30–31, 71, 132, 136, 146–147, 149
  role of grandchildren, 62, 124, 125–126
  role model, 109, 126
  role reversal, 105–106, 128
Clair, J.M., 21
Commonwealth Fund, 2
Coping
  strategies, 28–30, 33, 37, 40, 47, 52, 106–110, 118, 125, 155
  stress and coping theory, 8
  See also Educational programs, Religion, Respite, Social support
Coverman, S., 7
Coward, R.T., 4, 92

Dementia, See Alzheimer's disease
Demographic changes, See Male caregivers
Doctor relations, 21–22
Doty, P., 2
Driving privileges, 57, 98, 106, 108, 110
Dulac, G., 5
Duty, See Caregiving
Dwyer, J.W., 4, 92

Eastham, J., 2
Educational programs
    for caregivers, 80–82, 125, 159–164,
        193–204, 213–215
    for friends, 65, 83–84
    for professionals, 82–83
Elder abuse, 174–175

Farran, C.J., 8
Finley, N.J., 92
Fitting, M., 2, 3
Fontana, A., 12
Frankel, V.E., 8
Frey, J.H., 12
Fulmer, T.T., 174

George, L.K., 2, 3
Gilhooly, M.L.M., 2
Gilligan, C., 6
Glaser, B., 13
Godkin, M.A., 175
Gwyther, L., 3

Haley, W.E., 21
Harris, P.B., 1, 2, 3, 77, 86
Harrison, J., 5
Health care professionals
    reactions of, 131, 145–146
    See also Doctor relations, Social support-
        Alzheimer's association
Himes, C.L., 6
Hinrichsen, G.A., 171
Hoffman, C., 1
Home help services, 193–204
Hope, 22, 58
    See also Caregiving-hope
Horowitz, A., 1, 2, 3
Hudson, M.F., 175
Husband caregivers
    previous studies of, 1–3
    proportion of caregiving population, 2
    types of
        going it together, 53–63
        labor of love, 39–46
        men in transition, 63–71
        sense of duty, 46–53
        worker, 35–38
    See also Male caregivers

Johnsen, P.T., 1
Johnson, C.L., 2, 3, 94, 172
Johnson, T.F., 175

Kahana, E., 2
Kamo, Y., 4
Kaye, L.W., 1, 7
Kleban, M.H., 1
Kosberg, J.I., 5
Kupferer, S., 8

Lee, G.R., 4, 92
Legal/financial planning, See Alzheimer's
    disease
Levin, J.S., 172
Lincoln, C.E., 172
Loss, See Caregiving-loss
Lowe, B., 1
Lucas, M.J., 2

Male caregivers
    demographic changes, 4–8
    gender roles, 5–6, 25, 156, 170
    proportion in population, 1
    purpose of study, 8–9
    tasks/new roles, 27–28, 25, 38, 47,
        50, 91, 128
    See also Husband caregivers, Son
        caregivers
Mamiya, L.H., 172
McFadden, S.H., 8, 92
McKinlay, J.B., 3
Meaning of caregiving, See Caregiving
Miller, B., 2, 3
Montgomery, R., 4, 74
Motenko, A.K., 1, 2, 3
Mui, A.C., 2

Nursing home
    placement, 41, 93–94, 113, 120–121
    See also Residential settings

Oakley, A. 12
O'Neil, J.M., 5, 6
Osgood, N.J., 83

Pearlin, L.I., 8
Pillemer, K.A., 175

Racial differences, See Caregiving
Raminez, M., 171
Religion
    as a coping strategy, 42, 47, 62, 107–
        108, 114, 134
    African American and white differ-
        ences, 171–172
Residential settings

Alzheimer's care, 209–211
Respite
  as a coping strategy, 29, 40, 84
  services, 19, 84–85, 166, 193–204, 205–208
Roberts, D., 92
Rossiter, C.M., 74
Ruddick, S., 6

Salloway, S., 8
Sangl, J., 2, 3
Saulsberry, K., 21
Scharlach, A., 1
Schneider, B., 1
Schooler, C.E., 8
Schultz, R., 8
Shanas, E., 1
Sheley, J., 7
Siblings, role of, 92–93, 103–104, 114, 115–116, 120–121, 129, 132–133, 144, 148, 150, 152
Smyth, K.A., 77
Social class, 171–172
Social isolation, See Caregiving
Social support
  Alzheimer's association, 118–119, 120, 156
  friends, 45, 55, 118
  See also Children; Siblings; Son caregivers-role of wives; Support groups
Solomon, K., 5
Son caregivers
  previous studies of, 3–4, 92–94
  proportion of population, 3
  role model for, 109, 126
  role of wives, 107, 117, 118, 147, 148–149, 154–155
  types of
    dutiful son, 111–126
    going the extra mile, 127–141
    sharing the care, 148–157

strategic planners, 141–148
  See also Male caregivers
Steinmetz, S.K., 175
Stoller, E.P., 2, 4
Stone, R., 2, 3
Strauss, A., 13
Strieb, G.F., 1
Sullivan, L.M., 3
Support groups, 20, 41–42, 45, 74–79, 139
  computer networks, 77–78, 165, 191–192
  early stage, 49, 58, 69, 75–77, 187–190
  friendship clubs, 78–79
  male, 40, 75

Tatara, T., 174
Tatro, C., 6
Taylor, R.J., 172
Tennstedt, S.L., 3
Todd, P.A., 3
Toseland, R.W., 74

U.S. Bureau of the Census, 6, 7
U.S. Senate Special Committee on Aging, 1

Vinick, B.H., 3

Weinstein, G.W., 2
Wolf, R.S., 175
Work
  coping stategy, 107
  flexibility, 104–105, 110, 118
Wright, L.K., 3

Young, R.F., 2

Zarit, J.M., 3
Zarit, S., 3